This book is dedicated to the many male patients whom I have treated over the past 19 years. Most, if not all, of the questions contained herein were raised by them during the course of their diagnosis, treatment, and follow-up visits. Their quest for knowledge to better understand their urologic condition has prompted me to write this book. Their treatment, successes, and failures have highlighted the importance of painting a realistic picture of the various urologic conditions and their management. Making decisions and dealing with adverse outcomes requires knowledge—knowledge is power! This book is written to provide other men faced with similar urologic problems with the knowledge to actively participate in the decision-making regarding their urologic conditions. Changes in Medicare and proposed future changes in the healthcare system underscore the need for patients to take a more active role in their health care. Prostate cancer, benign prostatic hyperplasia (BPH), and sexual dysfunction are all conditions with a prevalence that increases with age. I thank my current and prior male patients who were treated for these conditions for providing me with the impetus to write this book, so that men faced with such conditions in the future will have a resource to assist them.

Contents

PART ONE

Prostate Cancer

What is the prostate gland and what does it do?

What are the warning signs of prostate cancer?

What options do I have for treatment of my prostate cancer?

More . . .

1. What is the prostate gland and what does it do?

The prostate gland is actually not a single gland. It is comprised of a collection of glands that are covered by a capsule. A **gland** is a structure or organ that produces a substance used in another part of the body. The prostate gland lies below the bladder, encircles the **urethra**, and lies in front of the rectum. Because it lies just in front of the rectum, the **posterior** aspect of the prostate can be assessed during a rectal examination. The normal size of the prostate gland is about the size of a walnut (**Figures 1 and 2**).

The prostate gland is divided into several *zones*, or areas. These divisions are based on locations of the tissue, but they also have some significance with respect

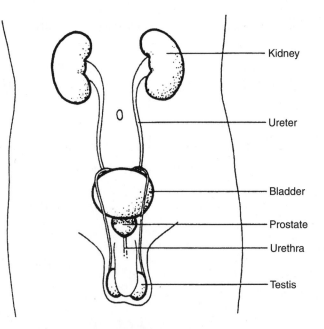

Figure 1   Anatomy of the male genitourinary system.

From *Prostate and Cancer* by Sheldon H.F. Marks. Copyright © 1995 by Sheldon Marks. Reprinted with permission of Perseus Books Publishers, a member of Perseus Books, LLC.

Gland

A structure or organ that produces substances that affect other areas of the body.

Urethra

The tube that runs from the bladder neck to the tip of the penis through which urine passes.

Posterior

The rear or back side.

The prostate gland is divided into several zones, or areas.

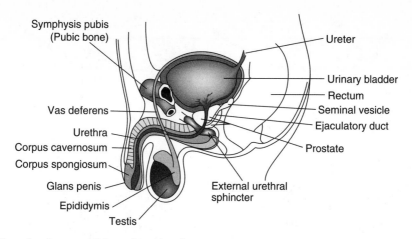

Figure 2   Anatomy of the male genitourinary system.

to benign prostatic hypertrophy (BPH) and prostate cancer. The zones are the transition zone, the peripheral zone, and the central zone (**Figure 3**). In most prostate cancers, the tumor occurs in the peripheral zone. In a few cases, the tumor is mostly located in the transition zone, around the urethra or toward the **abdomen**. In 85% of patients, the prostate cancer is **multifocal**, meaning that it is found in more than one area in the prostate. Seventy percent of prostate cancer patients with a **palpable** nodule, one that can be felt by a rectal examination, have cancer on the other side also. Another way to describe the prostate gland is to divide it into lobes. The prostate gland has five lobes: two lateral lobes, a middle lobe, an anterior lobe, and a posterior lobe. **Benign** (noncancerous) enlargement of the prostate typically occurs in the lateral lobes and may also affect the middle lobe.

The prostate gland contributes substances to the ejaculate that serve as nutrients to sperm. The prostate gland has a high amount of zinc in it. The reason for this is not clear, but it appears to help in fighting off infections.

Abdomen

The part of the body below the ribs and above the pelvic bone that contains organs such as the intestines, the liver, the kidneys, the stomach, the bladder, and the prostate.

Multifocal

Found in more than one area.

Palpable

Capable of being felt during a physical examination by an experienced doctor. In the case of prostate cancer, this refers to an abnormality of the prostate that can be felt during a rectal examination.

Benign

A growth that is not cancerous.

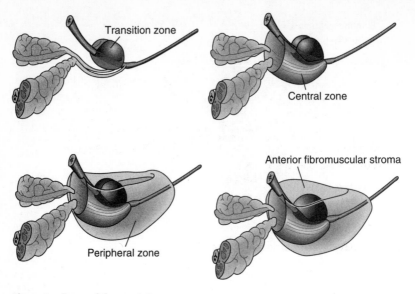

Figure 3   Zones of the prostate.

2. What are the signs and symptoms of an enlarged prostate (either cancer related or benign)?

The prostate gland in the adult male is normally about 20 to 25 cm³ in size.

Benign prostatic hyperplasia (BPH)

Noncancerous enlargement of the prostate.

The prostate gland in the adult male is normally about 20 to 25 cm^3 in size. Over time, the prostate gland may grow as a result of benign enlargement of the prostate, known as **benign prostatic hyperplasia (BPH)**, or as a result of prostate cancer. Enlargement of the prostate gland may cause changes in urinary symptoms; however, the severity of urinary symptoms does not correlate with the size of the prostate. In fact, some men with mildly enlarged prostates (for example, 40 cm^3) may be more symptomatic than men with greatly enlarged (>100 cm³) prostate glands. The symptoms of an enlarged prostate are caused by the prostate's resistance to the outflow of urine and the bladder's response to this resistance. Common symptoms include:

- Getting up at night to urinate one or more times per night (**nocturia**).
- Urinating frequently (eight or more times per day).
- Feeling that you have to urinate, but when you attempt to, finding that it takes a while for the urine to come out (**hesitancy**).
- Straining or pushing to get your urine stream started and/or to maintain your stream.
- Dribbling urine near the completion of voiding.
- A urine stream that stops and starts during voiding (**intermittency**).
- Feeling of incomplete emptying after voiding such that you feel that you could void again shortly.

Nocturia

Awakening one or more times at night with the desire to void.

Hesitancy

A delay in the start of the urine stream during voiding.

Intermittency

An inability to complete voiding and emptying the bladder with one single contraction of the bladder. A stopping and starting of the urine stream during urination.

3. What is PSA? What is the normal PSA value? What is free total PSA?

PSA stands for prostate specific antigen. PSA is a chemical produced by prostate cells, both normal and cancerous. PSA is not produced significantly by other cells in the body. Normally, only a small amount of PSA gets into the bloodstream. However, when the prostate is irritated, inflamed, or damaged, such as in prostatitis and prostate cancer, PSA leaks into the bloodstream more easily, causing the level of PSA in the blood to be higher. The normal range is usually 0 to 4.0 ng/mL; however, in younger men a lower range is used (**Table 1**). The normal range for PSA varies with age and race.

Table 1 Age-Adjusted Normal PSA Ranges

Age (yr)	Normal range (ng/mL)
40–49	0–2.5 (0–2.0 for African Americans)
50–59	0–3.5
60–69	0–4.5
70–79	0–6.5

Reprinted with permission from Oesterling et al. *JAMA* 1993; 270:860–864. Copyright © American Medical Association.

PSA that is attached to chemicals (proteins) is bound PSA and PSA that is not attached to proteins is called free PSA.

Bound PSA

PSA attached to the proteins in the bloodstream.

Free PSA

The PSA present that is not bound to proteins. It is often expressed as a ratio of free PSA to total PSA in terms of percent, which is the free PSA divided by the total PSA × 100.

Once a baseline normal PSA has been obtained, the actual number becomes less important and the rate of change of the PSA over time becomes more important.

PSA is found in two forms in the bloodstream. PSA that is attached to chemicals (proteins) is **bound PSA** and PSA that is not attached to proteins is called **free PSA**. The amount of each form is measured, and a ratio of the free PSA to the free plus bound (or total) PSA is calculated.

The PSA present that is not bound to proteins is often expressed as a ratio of free PSA to total PSA. It's expressed as a percentage, which is the free PSA, divided by the total PSA × 100.

The higher this number, the less likely that prostate cancer is present. A free PSA value greater than 14–25%

suggests that the presence of prostate cancer is less likely. This ratio may be helpful in individuals with mildly elevated PSAs in the 4–10 ng/mL range for whom the doctor is deciding whether to perform a prostate biopsy.

PSA density refers to the PSA per gram of prostate tissue and is calculated by dividing the PSA by the calculated prostate volume in grams estimated by transrectal ultrasound. A PSA density > 0.15 is felt to be suggestive of prostate cancer.

PSA velocity refers to the change in PSA level over time. As men get older the prostate tends to enlarge, thus it is expected that the PSA may increase slightly over time. In men with a PSA < 4 ng/ml it is felt that a PSA velocity > 0.35 ng/ml is cause for concern, whereas in men with a total PSA > 4 ng/ml a PSA velocity of > 0.75 ng/ml is cause for concern for the risk of prostate cancer.

4. What causes the PSA to rise?

Anything that irritates or inflames the prostate can increase the PSA, such as a urinary tract infection, prostatitis, prostate stones, a recent urinary catheter or cystoscopy (a look into the bladder through a specialized telescope-like instrument), recent prostate biopsy, or prostate surgery. Sexual intercourse may increase the PSA up to 10%, and a vigorous rectal examination or prostatic massage before the PSA blood test is drawn may also increase the PSA. Benign enlargement of the prostate (BPH) may also increase the PSA because more prostate cells are present, thus more PSA is produced (see Question 3).

5. Are there medications that may affect the PSA? Does testosterone therapy cause the PSA to increase?

Yes, some medications can affect the PSA. Finasteride (Proscar) and Dutasteride (Avodart), medications used to shrink the prostate in men with benign enlargement of the prostate, decrease the PSA up to 50%. This decrease in PSA occurs predictably no matter what your initial PSA is. Any sustained increases in PSA while you are taking Proscar or Avodart (provided that you are taking the Proscar or Avodart regularly) should be evaluated. The percentage of free PSA (the amount of free PSA/the amount of total PSA) is not significantly decreased by these medications and should remain stable while you are taking Proscar or Avodart. Other medications that can decrease the amount of testosterone produced by your testicles, such as ketoconazole, may decrease the PSA. Decreasing the amount of testosterone may cause both benign and cancerous prostate tissue to shrink. Testosterone is broken down in the body to a chemical, dihydrotestosterone, which is responsible for the stimulation of prostate growth. Thus, the addition of testosterone may stimulate the growth of normal prostate cells and possibly prostate cancer cells. Because normal prostate cells produce PSA, it is not unreasonable to expect that an increase in the normal cells present in the prostate would lead to an increase in the PSA. Prostate cancer is composed of both hormone-sensitive and hormone-insensitive cells. The hormone-insensitive cells grow regardless of the availability of testosterone or its breakdown products, whereas the hormone-sensitive cells appear to be dependent on the male hormone for growth. Thus, the addition of testosterone may affect the growth of these hormone-sensitive cells. Testosterone therapy

Prostate cancer is composed of both hormone-sensitive and hormone-insensitive cells.

has not been shown to cause the development of prostate cancer.

6. Are there any other blood tests to check for prostate cancer?

Early Prostate Cancer Antigen (EPCA) and EPCA-2 have been demonstrated to be plasma-based markers for prostate cancer. EPCA is found throughout the prostate and represents a field effect associated with prostate cancer, whereas, EPCA-2 is found only in the prostate cancer tissue. However, EPCA-2 is able to get into the plasma, the liquid part of the blood, allowing for it to be detected by a blood test. In preliminary studies, EPCA-2 has been able to identify men with prostate cancer who had normal PSA levels. This data, however, is preliminary and further studies are needed to validate the sensitivity and specificity of these markers. Others are investigating the ability for urinary markers to detect prostate cancer, specifically alpha-methyl-acyl-CoA racemase (AMACR) and prostate cancer antigen 3 (PCA 3) urinary transcript levels obtained from urine sediments following digital rectal examination and prostatic massage.

7. What is prostate cancer?

Prostate cancer is a malignant growth of the glandular cells of the prostate. Our body is composed of billions of **cells**; they are the smallest unit in the body. Normally, each cell functions for a while, then dies and is replaced in an organized manner. This results in the appropriate number of cells being present to carry out necessary cell functions. Sometimes there can be an uncontrolled replacement of cells, leaving the cells unable to organize as they did before. Such abnormal growth of cells is called a **tumor**. Tumors may be benign (noncancerous)

Prostate cancer is a malignant growth of the glandular cells of the prostate.

Cells

The smallest unit of the body. Tissues in the body are made up of cells.

Tumor

Abnormal tissue growth that may be cancerous or non-cancerous (benign).

Cancer

Abnormal and uncontrolled growth of cells in the body that may spread, injure areas of the body, and lead to death.

Malignancy

Cancer: uncontrolled growth of cells that can spread to other areas of the body and cause death.

Lymph

A clear fluid that is found throughout the body. Lymph fluid helps fight infections.

Lymph node(s)

Small bean-shaped glands that are found throughout the body. Lymph fluid passes through the lymph nodes, which filter out bacteria, cancer cells, and toxic chemicals.

or malignant (cancerous). **Cancer** is abnormal cell growth and disorder such that the cancer cells can grow without the normal controls and limits. A **malignancy** is a cancerous growth that has the potential to spread and cause damage to other tissues of the body or even lead to death. Cancers can spread locally into surrounding tissues, or cancer cells can break away from the tumor and enter body fluids, such as the blood and lymph, and spread to other parts of the body. **Lymph** is an almost clear fluid that drains waste from cells. This fluid travels in vessels to the **lymph nodes**, small bean-shaped structures that filter unwanted substances, such as cancer cells and bacteria, out of the fluid. Lymph nodes may become filled with cancer cells.

As with most cancers, prostate cancer is not contagious.

8. How common is prostate cancer?

There are more than 100 different types of cancer. In the United States, a man has a 50% chance of developing some type of cancer in his lifetime. In American men, (excluding skin cancer) prostate cancer is the most common cancer. Prostate cancer accounts for about 33% (234,460) of cases of cancer (**Table 2**). More than 75% of the cases of prostate cancer are diagnosed in men older than 65 years. Based on cases diagnosed between 1995 and 2001, it is estimated that 91% of the new cases of prostate cancer are expected to be diagnosed at local or regional stages (see staging of prostate cancer), for which 5-year survival is nearly 100%. It is estimated that prostate cancer will be the cause of death in 9% of men, 27,350 prostate cancer related deaths. In the United States, deaths from prostate cancer have decreased significantly by 4.1% per year from 1994 to 2004. Most notably, the death rate for African American men in the United States has decreased by 6%.

Table 2   Cancer Statistics for Men in the United States—2006

Cancer Site	Estimated % of All New Cancer Diagnoses	Estimated Number of New Cases
Prostate	33%	234,460
Digestive system	10%	72,800
Lung and bronchus	13%	92,700

Reprinted with permission from Ahnedub GM, Suegek RM, Ward E et al. Cancer Statistics, 2006. *CA Cancer J Clin* 2006;56:106–130 [published erratum appears in *CA Cancer J Clin* 2006;56:109].

9. What are the risk factors for prostate cancer, and who is at risk? Is there anything that decreases the risk of developing prostate cancer?

Theoretically, all men are at risk for developing prostate cancer. The prevalence of prostate cancer increases with age, and the increase with age is greater for prostate cancer than for any other cancer.

1:10,000   <39 years of age
1:103   40–59 years of age
1:8   60–79 years of age

Basically, every 10 years after the age of 40 years, the incidence of prostate cancer nearly doubles, with a risk of 10% for men in their 50s increasing to 70% for those in their 80s. However, in most older men, the prostate cancer does not grow and many die of other causes and are not identified as having prostate cancer before their death.

Prostate cancer is 66% more common among African Americans, and it is twice as likely to be fatal in African Americans as in Caucasians. However, blacks in Africa have one of the lowest rates of prostate cancer in the world. Males of Asian descent living in the United States

Theoretically, all men are at risk for developing prostate cancer.

Prostate Cancer

have lower rates of prostate cancer than Caucasians, but higher rates than Asian males in their native countries. Japan appears to have the lowest prostate cancer death rate, compared with Switzerland, which has the highest (**Figure 4**).

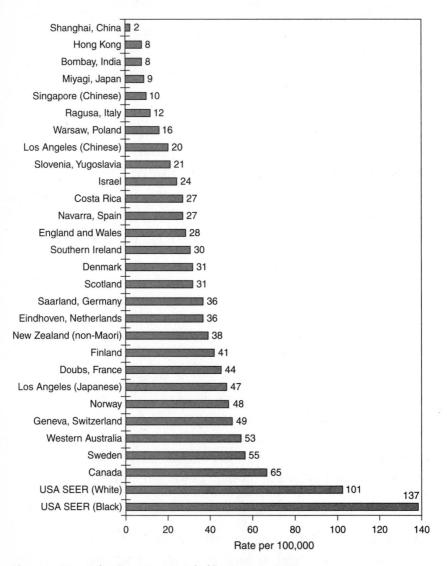

Figure 4   International prostate cancer incidence rates—1998.

Standford JL, Stephenson RA, Coyle LM et al. Prostate Cancer Trends 1973–1995. Bethesda, MD. Cancer Surveillence, Epidemiology, and End Results (SEER) Program, National Cancer Institute 1998.

Prostate cancer is related to sex hormones. Prostate cancer rarely develops in men who had their testicles removed (**castration**) at an early age. There is a correlation between prostate cancer and high levels of testosterone. There does not appear to be any clear correlation between body size and risk of prostate cancer but men with prostate cancer who had weight gain in early adulthood tend to have more aggressive cancers. Smoking does not appear to increase your risk of cancer, though smokers tend to have more aggressive cancer than nonsmokers. Physical activity appears to decrease the risk of prostate cancer.

Castration

The removal of both testicles.

The effects of vasectomy on the risk of prostate cancer are unclear.

The effects of vasectomy on the risk of prostate cancer are unclear. Some studies have demonstrated an increased risk of prostate cancer with vasectomy, but these individuals tended to have a lower grade, lower stage prostate cancer that is associated with a better prognosis. Other studies have failed to confirm an increased risk of prostate cancer after vasectomy. **Vasectomy** is the minor surgical sterilization procedure in which the **vas deferens** (the sperm duct) is cut and either clipped, tied, or cauterized to prevent it from reattaching itself. Vasectomy does not affect testosterone production or release of testosterone from the testicles into the bloodstream; it only prevents sperm from leaving the testis. Current medical wisdom holds that vasectomy does not increase your risk of prostate cancer.

Vasectomy

A procedure in which the vas deferens are cut and tied off, clipped, or cauterized to prevent the exit of sperm from the testicles. It makes a man sterile.

Vas deferens

A tiny tube that connects the testicles to the urethra through which sperm passes.

The Cancer Risk Calculator for Prostate Cancer has been developed as a tool to help identify one's risk of having prostate cancer. The calculator may be applied to men age 50 years or older, with no previous diagnosis of prostate cancer and DRE and PSA results less than 1 year old. The calculator may also be applied to men undergoing prostate cancer screening with PSA and

DRE, as it was developed from the Prostate Cancer Prevention Trial. The calculator is designed to provide a preliminary assessment of risk of prostate cancer if a prostate biopsy is performed. One can find the prostate cancer risk calculator online, either by searching for "cancer risk calculator for prostate cancer" or by going to the National Cancer Institute website and looking under early detection research network.

A recent study called the "Prostate Cancer Prevention Trial" (PCPT) demonstrated that finasteride (Proscar) at a dose of 5mg/day decreases the likelihood of developing prostate cancer by 26% when compared to placebo (sugar pill). In addition, finasteride decreased the risk of high grade PIN (which may be a precursor of prostate cancer) by about the same rate. In this study, finasteride lowered the PSA by 50% after 2 months of treatment.

"Asymptomatic men with a PSA < 3.0 ng/ml who are regularly screened with PSA or who are anticipating undergoing annual PSA screening for early detection of prostate cancer may benefit from a discussion of both the benefits of 5-alpha reductase inhibitors for 7 years for the prevention of prostate cancer and the potential risks (2–4% increase in reported erectile dysfunction and gynecomastia [enlarged and/or painful breasts], and decrease in ejaculate volume in those receiving finasteride in the study compared to those receiving placebo)."

www.auanet.org/content/guidelines-and-qualitycare/clinical-guidelines/main-reports/pcredinh.pdf.

Results of the "Reduction by Dutasteride of Prostate Cancer" (REDUCE) trial showed that the 5-alpha-reductase inhibitor dutasteride at doses of 0.5 mg/day decreased the relative risk of prostate cancer by 23% compared to placebo. Furthermore, the risk was markedly decreased in the number of high-grade tumors, with no absolute increase in incidence compared to placebo.

Dietary and genetic (hereditary) factors may also play a role in the risk of developing cancer.

Familial-Related Risks

In certain cases, it appears that the risk for prostate cancer is passed on to males in the family. The younger the family member is when he is diagnosed with prostate cancer, the higher the risk is for male relatives to have prostate cancer at a younger age. The risk also increases with the number of relatives affected with prostate cancer (**Table 3**).

Gene-Related Risks

It is thought that 9% of all prostate cancers, and more than 40% of prostate cancers occurring in younger males,

In certain cases, it appears that the risk for prostate cancer is passed on to males in the family. The younger the family member is when he is diagnosed with prostate cancer, the higher the risk is for male relatives to have prostate cancer at a younger age.

Table 3   Relative Risk for Prostate Cancer with Affected Relatives

Age of Onset (Years)	Additional Relatives Beyond One First-Degree Relative Affected	Relative Risk
70	None	1.0
60	None	1.4
50	None	2.0
70	One or more	4.0
60	One or more	5.0
50	One or more	7.0

Reprinted with permission from Carter BS, Bovea GS, Beaty TH et al. *J Urol* 1993;150:797–802.

are related to genetic causes. Abnormalities of genes of chromosomes 1 and the X chromosome are associated with an increased risk of prostate cancer. One such gene, the HPC1 gene, appears to cause about one third of all inherited cases of prostate cancer. There also appears to be a gene that is carried on the X chromosome (the chromosome passed on to the male by his mother) that may increase the risk of prostate cancer. This X chromosome related increased risk of prostate cancer might somehow play a part in the identification of a higher incidence of prostate cancer in male relatives of women with breast cancer.

Ethnicity–Related Risks

Black men are more likely to get prostate cancer at a younger age, and they often have a more aggressive cancer. Of all population groups in the world, African American men have the highest rate of prostate cancer. The reason for this is not known. Because they are at higher risk, African American men should start prostate cancer screening at a younger age than Caucasian men.

African American men should start prostate cancer screening at a younger age than Caucasian men.

Diet–Related Risks

A variety of dietary risk factors exist for prostate cancer. Several studies suggest that a high-fat diet stimulates prostate cancer to grow. In particular, beef and high-fat dairy products appear to be stimulators of prostate cancer. Conversely, a low-fat diet rich in fruits and vegetables may help decrease the risk of prostate cancer. Such healthful foods include soy (tofu and soy milk), tomatoes, green tea, red grapes, strawberries, raspberries, blueberries, peas, watermelon, rosemary, garlic, and citrus. Soy contains substances called phytoestrogens, which resemble the female sex hormone estrogen. In dietary-doses—that is, amounts normally found in foods, not the amounts in supplements—phytoestrogens can decrease the risk of prostate cancer. Green tea contains **antioxidants**, which are chemicals that help prevent changes in cells and reduce damage that can cause the cells to become cancerous.

Vitamin E is a free radical scavenger and is also associated with a decreased risk of prostate cancer, but men with a history of bleeding problems or who take blood thinners should discuss the use of vitamin E with their doctor before taking it.

A high intake of dairy products has also been associated with an increased risk of prostate cancer.

Vitamin D deficiency has been associated with an increased risk of prostate cancer.

High levels of fructose, a form of sugar, have been associated with a lower risk of prostate cancer. Selenium has been associated with a decreased risk of prostate cancer. Lycopene, a carotenoid (chemicals that give orange, red, or yellow coloring to plants), is associated with a decreased risk of prostate cancer. Lycopene is found in high levels in tomatoes and is beneficial only if one eats cooked tomatoes, such as tomato sauce, not tomato juice. Many studies are in the process of looking at the effects of such dietary risks.

10. What are the warning signs of prostate cancer?

Prostate cancer gives no typical warning signs that it is present in your body. It often grows very slowly, and some of the symptoms related to enlargement of the prostate are typical of noncancerous enlargement of the prostate, known as benign prostatic hyperplasia (BPH).

Antioxidant

A chemical that helps prevent changes in cells and reduce damage to the cell that can cause it to become cancerous.

Prostate Cancer

With more advanced disease, you may have fatigue, weight loss, and generalized aches and pains.

When the disease has spread to the bones, it may cause pain in the area. Bone pain may present in different ways. In some men, it may cause continuous pain, while in others, the pain may be intermittent. It may be confined to a particular area of the body or move around the body; it may be variable during the day and respond differently to rest and activity. If there is significant weakening of the bone(s), fractures may occur. More common sites of bone metastases include the hips, back, ribs, and shoulders. Some of these sites are also common locations for arthritis, so the presence of pain in any of these areas is not definitive for prostate cancer.

If prostate cancer spreads locally to the lymph nodes, it often does not cause any symptoms. Rarely, if there is extensive lymph node involvement, leg swelling may occur.

In patients with advanced cancer that has spread to the spine, paralysis can occur if the nerves are compressed because of either collapse of the spine or tumor growing into the spine.

Ureters

Tubes that connect the kidneys to the bladder, through which urine passes into the bladder.

If the prostate cancer grows into the floor (bottom) of the bladder, or if a large amount of cancer is present in the pelvic lymph nodes, one or both **ureters** can be obstructed. Signs and symptoms of ureteral obstruction include decreased urine volume, no urine volume if both ureters are blocked, back pain, nausea, vomiting, and possibly fevers if infections occur.

Blood in the urine and blood in the ejaculate are usually not related to prostate cancer; however, if these are present, you should seek urologic evaluation.

In individuals with widespread metastatic disease, bleeding problems can occur. In addition, patients with prostate cancer may develop anemia. The anemia may be related to extensive tumor in the bone, hormonal therapy, or the length of time you have had the cancer. Because the blood count tends to drop slowly, you may not have any symptoms of anemia. Some individuals with very significant anemia may have weakness, orthostatic hypotension (lowering of the blood pressure when you stand up), dizziness, shortness of breath, and the feeling of being ill and tired. Symptoms of advanced disease and their treatments are listed in **Table 4**.

Blood in the urine and blood in the ejaculate are usually not related to prostate cancer.

Prostate Cancer

11. What causes prostate cancer? What causes prostate cancer to grow?

The exact causes of prostate cancer are not known. Prostate cancer may develop because of changes in genes. Alterations in androgen (male hormone) related genes have been associated with an increased risk of cancer. Alterations in genes may be caused by environmental factors, such as diet. The more abnormal the gene, the higher is the likelihood of developing prostate cancer. In rare cases, prostate cancer may be inherited. In such cases, 88% of the individuals will have prostate cancer by the age of 85 years. Males who have a particular gene, the breast cancer mutation (BRCA1), have a threefold higher risk of developing prostate cancer than do other men. Changes in a certain chromosome, p53, in prostate cancer are associated with high-grade aggressive prostate cancer.

Table 4   Common Symptom-Directed Treatment Strategies in Advanced Prostate Cancer

Symptom	Treatment

Bone pain	Irradiation
	   Localized metastasis: external beam
	   Widespread metastasis: total body irradiation;
	     intravenous infusion
	Bisphosphonates
	   Zoledronic acid alendronate, neridronate
	   Intravenous/intravenous + oral
	Steroids
	   Oral prednisone
	Chemotherapy
	   Mitoxantrone
	   Investigational regime: taxotere/estramustine
	Analgesics
	   NSAIDs
	   Narcotic agents

Bone fracture	Surgical stabilization
Bladder obstruction	Hormonal treatment Transurethral prostatectomy Repeated debulking transurethral resections Alum irrigation Urethral catheter balloon intervention ($\leq$ 24 hr) Surgery
Ureteral obstruction	Endocrine therapy Radiation therapy Percutaneous nephrostomy Indwelling ureteral stents
Spinal cord compression	Intravenous and/or oral steroids Posterior laminectomy Radiation therapy
Dissemination intravascular coagulation (DIC)	Intravenous heparin and EACA Supplementation (e.g., platelets, fresh whole blood, packed erythrocytes, frozen plasma, or cryoprecipitate)
Anemia	Iron and vitamin supplementation Bone marrow stimulants (e.g., erythropoietin) Transfusion therapy
Edema	Compression stockings Leg elevation Diuretics

EACA, epsilon aminocaproic acid; NSAIDs, nonsteroidal anti-inflammatory drugs.

From Smith JA et al. *Urology* 1999; 54(suppl 6A):8–14. Reprinted with permission from Elsevier Science.

Prostate cancer, similar to breast cancer, is hormone sensitive. Prostate cancer growth is stimulated by the male hormones testosterone and dihydrotestosterone (a chemical that the body makes from testosterone). Testosterone is responsible for many normal changes, both physical and behavioral, that occur in a man's life, such as voice change and hair growth. The testis makes almost 90% of the testosterone in the body. A small amount of testosterone is made by the **adrenal glands** (a paired set of glands found above the kidneys that produce a variety of substances and hormones that are essential for daily living). In the bones, a chemical called transferrin, which is made by the liver and stored in the bones, also appears to stimulate the growth of prostate cancer cells. When cancers develop, they secrete chemicals that cause blood vessels to grow into the cancer and bring nutrients to the cancer so that it can grow.

12. Where does prostate cancer spread?

As the prostate cancer grows, it grows through the prostate, the prostate capsule, and the fat that surrounds the prostate capsule. Because the prostate gland lies below the bladder and attaches to it, the prostate cancer can also grow up into the base of the bladder.

Prostate cancer can also grow into the **seminal vesicles**, which are located adjacent to the prostate. It may continue to grow locally in the pelvis into muscles within the pelvis; into the rectum, which lies behind the prostate; or into the sidewall of the pelvis. The spread of cancer to other sites is called metastasis. When prostate cancer spreads outside of the capsule and the fatty tissue, it usually goes to two main areas in the body: the lymph nodes that drain the prostate and the bones. The more commonly involved lymph nodes are those in the pelvis (**Figure 5**), and bones that are more

Prostate cancer, similar to breast cancer, is hormone sensitive.

Prostate Cancer

Adrenal glands
Glands located above each kidney. These glands produce several different hormones, including sex hormones.

Seminal vesicles
Glandular structures that are located above and behind the prostate. They produce fluid that is part of the ejaculate.

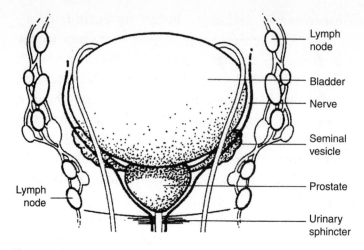

Figure 5   Lymph node drainage from the prostate.

From *Prostate and Cancer* by Sheldon H.F. Marks. Copyright © 1995 by Sheldon Marks. Reprinted with permission of Perseus Books Publishers, a member of Perseus Books, LLC.

commonly affected are the spine (backbones) and the ribs. Less commonly, prostate cancer can spread to solid organs in the body, such as the liver.

13. What is prostate cancer screening?

The goal of any screening is to evaluate populations of people in an effort to diagnose the disease early.

The goal of any screening is to evaluate populations of people in an effort to diagnose the disease early. Thus, the goal of prostate cancer screening is the early detection of prostate cancer, ideally at the curable stage. Prostate cancer screening includes both a digital rectal examination and a serum PSA. Each of these is important in the screening process, and an abnormality in either warrants further evaluation. Only about 25% of prostate cancers are revealed by rectal examination; most are detected by an abnormal PSA. Some studies suggest that even with PSA-based prostate cancer screening, up to 15% of men will have undetected prostate cancer. Newer screening tools, such as EPCA and EPCA-2, are being investigated (see Question 6).

Because the prostate gland lies in front of the rectum, the back wall of the prostate gland can be felt by putting a gloved, lubricated finger into the rectum and feeling the prostate by pressing on the anterior wall of the rectum (**Figure 6**). The rectal examination allows one to feel only the back of the prostate. Ideally, the same doctor should perform the rectal examination each year so that the doctor is able to detect subtle changes in your prostate. The exam can be performed by an urologist or by an experienced primary care provider. If the primary care provider is concerned about your examination, you will be referred to a urologist. On rectal examination, the examiner is checking the prostate for a nodule. A prostate nodule is a firm, hard area in the prostate that feels like the knuckle of your finger. A prostate nodule may be cancerous and should be biopsied, but not all prostate nodules are cancers. Other causes of a nodule

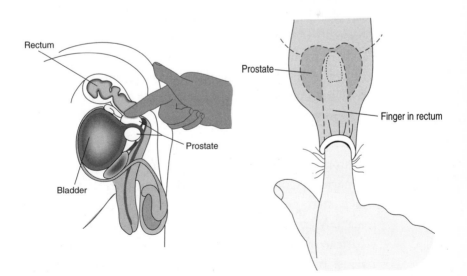

Figure 6   Digital rectal examination of the prostate.

or a firm area in the prostate include prostatitis (prostate infection or inflammation), prostate calculi, an old **infarct** in the prostate, or abnormalities of the rectum, such as a hemorrhoid. If you have had your rectum removed, then your doctor will rely on the PSA. If the PSA were to rise significantly, then a prostate biopsy would be performed. A transrectal ultrasound biopsy likewise cannot be performed in individuals without a rectum. In this situation, the biopsy is performed transperineally, which means through the perineum (the area under the scrotum). Performing biopsies in this way can be more uncomfortable, and they are often performed with some form of anesthesia (general, spinal, or intravenous sedation).

Prostate cancer screening should be performed on a yearly basis, except for men with a very low initial PSA level who may want to consider screening every other year. As you continue with screening on a yearly basis, changes in the PSA (beyond what is believed to be a change caused by benign growth of the prostate) or rectal examination will prompt further evaluation. It is hoped that, through the use of prostate cancer screening, the morbidity and mortality associated with prostate cancer will be diminished. More recent studies are showing increased survival as a result of prostate cancer screening.

Historically, the American Urologic Association and the American College of Surgeons recommend that most men start prostate cancer screening at the age of 50 years. Men with a family history of prostate cancer and African Americans should begin screening at age 40 years. In April 2009, the American Urologic Association issued new guidelines lowering the age for beginning

Infarct

An area of dead tissue resulting from a sudden loss of its blood supply.

prostate-specific antigen (PSA) and digital rectal examination (DRE) screening to 40 years for relatively healthy, well-informed men who wanted to be tested.

Prostate cancer screening is of maximal benefit for men who are going to live long enough to experience the benefits of treatment, typically, survival for at least 10 years from the diagnosis of prostate cancer. Thus, if you have medical conditions that make survival of 10 additional years less likely, you probably would not benefit from the early detection and treatment of prostate cancer and could stop prostate cancer screening. In addition, if you feel that you would not want any treatment for prostate cancer regardless of your age and overall health, then you should stop prostate cancer screening.

A combination of PSA and a digital rectal examination is the best screening for prostate cancer.

14. What does a TRUS guided prostate biopsy involve?

The transrectal ultrasound may be performed in your urologist's office or in the radiology department, depending on your institution. In preparation for the study, you may be asked to take an enema to clean stool out of the rectum and to take some antibiotics around the time of the study. You will be asked to stop taking any aspirin or nonsteroidal anti-inflammatory medications, such as ibuprofen (Motrin or Advil) for about 1 week prior to the biopsy to minimize bleeding. The doctor will ask you to lie on your side with your legs bent and brought up to your abdomen. The ultrasound probe, which is a little larger than your thumb, is then gently placed into the rectum. This can cause some transient discomfort that usually stops when the probe is in place and completely goes away when the probe is removed. Men who have had prior rectal surgery, who have active hemorrhoids, or who are very anxious and cannot relax the external sphincter muscle may have more discomfort. Once the probe is in a good position, the prostate will be evaluated to make sure that there are no suspicious areas on the ultrasound. Ultrasound looks at tissues by sound waves. The probe emits the sound waves, and the waves hit the prostate and are bounced off the prostate and surrounding tissue. The waves then return to the ultrasound probe, and a picture is developed on the screen. The sound waves do not cause any discomfort. Prostate cancer tends to cause less reflection of the sound waves, a trait referred to as **hypoechoic**, so the area often looks different in an ultrasound image than the normal prostate tissue. After the prostate has been evaluated, biopsies are obtained. The transrectal ultrasound allows the urologist to visualize the location for the biopsies. A minimum of six to eight biopsies are obtained and more frequently twelve. These biopsies are distributed between the top, the bottom, and the middle aspect of the prostate on each side. If you have a large prostate gland, have suspicious areas on ultrasound, or have had prior negative prostate biopsies, more biopsies may be obtained.

Side effects of TRUS guided prostate biopsy include transient discomfort related to the ultrasound probe, the needle guide, and the biopsy itself. After the TRUS biopsy one may experience blood in the urine, the semen (ejaculate), and/or in the stools. A urinary tract infection and/or acute prostatitis may occur and would present with frequency of urination, burning, and perineal discomfort and, in some cases, a fever.

Hypoechoic

In ultrasonography, giving off few echoes; said of tissues or structures that reflect relatively few ultrasound waves directed at them.

15. Are all prostate cancers the same? Are there different grades?

Not all prostate cancers are the same. Prostate cancers may vary in the grade of the cancer and the stage of the cancer.

The grade of a cancer is a term used to describe how the cancer cells look. That is, whether the cells look aggressive and not very similar to normal cells (high grade) or whether they look very similar to normal cells (low grade). The grade of the cancer is an important factor in predicting long-term results of treatment, response to treatment, and survival. With prostate cancer, the most commonly used grading system is the **Gleason scale**. In this grading system, cells are examined by a pathologist under the microscope and assigned a number based on how the cancer cells look and how they are arranged together (**Figure 7**). Because prostate cancer may be composed of cancer cells of different grades, the pathologist assigns numbers to the two predominant grades present. The numbers range from 1 (low grade) to 5 (high grade). Typically, the Gleason score is the total of these two numbers; for example, a man with a Gleason grade of 2 and 3 in his prostate cancer would have a Gleason score of 5. An exception to this occurs where the highest (most aggressive) pattern present in a biopsy is neither the most predominant nor the second most predominant pattern. In this situation, the Gleason score is obtained by combining the most predominant pattern grade with the highest grade. Occasionally, if a small component of a tumor on prostatectomy is of a pattern that is higher than the two most predominant patterns, then the minor component is noted as a tertiary grade to the pathology report.

The grade of a cancer is a term used to describe how the cancer cells look.

Gleason grade

A commonly used method to classify how cells appear in cancerous prostate tissues; the less the cancerous cells look like normal cells, the more malignant the cancer; two numbers, each from 1 to 5, are assigned to the two most predominant types of cells present. These two numbers are added together to produce the Gleason score. Higher numbers indicate more aggressive cancers.

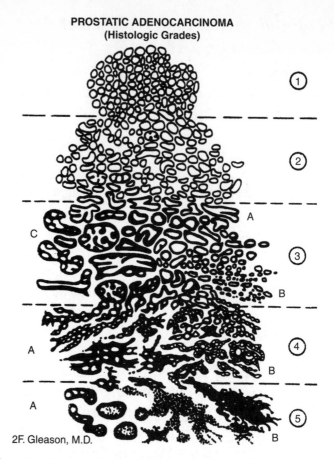

PROSTATIC ADENOCARCINOMA
(Histologic Grades)

2F. Gleason, M.D.

Figure 7   Gleason grading system of prostate adenocarcinoma.

Reprinted with permission from JI Epstein, *Campbell's Urology*, (7th Ed). Copyright © 1997 W.B. Saunders Co.

Low score cancers are those with a Gleason score of 2, 3, or 4. Intermediate score cancers are those with a Gleason score of 5, 6, or 7. And high score cancers are those with a Gleason score of 8, 9, or 10. The speed of growth and the aggressiveness of the cancer increase with the Gleason score. Gleason scores 8 through 10 are highly aggressive tumors and are often difficult to cure.

Sometimes these cancers are so abnormal that they do not even produce PSA. The grade of the cancer

Sometimes these cancers are so abnormal that they do not even produce PSA.

identified by the biopsies may differ from the grade that is present in the entire prostate because it is possible that the biopsy may not identify areas of higher-grade cancers.

Other abnormalities that may be noted on the biopsy result are PIN and atypical glands. **PIN, or prostatic intraepithelial neoplasia,** is identified by the pathologist examining the prostate biopsies. PIN has been thought to be a precancerous lesion. More recently, PIN has been divided into two types, low-grade PIN and high-grade PIN, based on how the cells look. Low-grade PIN does not appear to have any increased risk of prostate cancer. High-grade PIN, however, is often found in association with prostate cancer. In 35–45% of men who undergo a repeat biopsy for high-grade PIN, prostate cancer cells are present in the repeat biopsy. If your doctor has performed multiple biopsies (i.e., 10–12) then the recommendation is to consider a delayed repeat biopsy. If your doctor only did six biopsies, then an immediate repeat biopsy is indicated. "Atypical gland; suspicious for cancer" is noted on the pathology report when the pathologist sees an atypical area that has most of the features of cancer, but a definitive diagnosis of cancer cannot be made due to the small size of the area and the small number of abnormal cells present. Repeat biopsy in patients with this diagnosis have up to a 60% chance of having prostate cancer present in a repeat biopsy. Thus, the finding of atypical gland; suspicious for cancer warrants an immediate rebiopsy (within 3 months) with increased number of biopsies from the abnormal area and the areas nearby. If no cancer is found on the repeat biopsy then close follow-up with PSA, digital rectal examination, and periodic biopsy may be needed. See www.pccnc.org/early.

PIN (prostatic intraepithelial neoplasia)

An abnormal area in a prostate biopsy specimen that is not cancerous, but may become cancerous or be associated with cancer elsewhere in the prostate.

16. What is prostate cancer staging?

By staging your cancer, your doctor is trying to assess, based on your prostate biopsy results, your physical examination, your PSA, and other tests and X-rays (if obtained), whether your prostate cancer is confined to the prostate, and if it is not, to what extent it has spread. Studies of large numbers of men who have undergone radical prostatectomy and pelvic lymph node dissections have provided for the development of nomograms predicting the pathologic stage of CaP based on clinical stage (TNM), PSA, and Gleason score (**Table 5**). It was initially thought that magnetic resonance imaging (MRI) would be very helpful in determining whether capsular penetration and extracapsular disease were present; however, it has only proved to be useful in centers that perform large numbers of MRIs. Similarly, the use of computed tomographic (CT) scanning in assessing whether or not the cancer has spread to the pelvic lymph nodes has been disappointing.

Knowing the stage (the size and the extent of spread) of the prostate cancer helps the doctor counsel you on treatment options. Your doctor may tell you a clinical stage (**Figure 8**), based on your rectal examination, prostate biopsies, and radiographic/nuclear medicine studies (CT scan, bone scan, MRI). Pathological staging is performed when a pathologist examines the prostate, seminal vesicles, and pelvic lymph nodes (if removed) at the time of radical prostatectomy. The most common staging system used is called the **TNM System**. In this system, T refers to the size of the tumor in the prostate, N refers to the extent of cancerous involvement of the lymph nodes, and M refers to the presence or absence of metastases (deposits of prostate cancer outside of the

---

Knowing the stage (the size and the extent of spread) of the prostate cancer helps the doctor counsel you on treatment options.

TNM system

Tumor, nodes, and metastases. The most common staging system for prostate cancer.

Table 5   Nomograms Predicting Pathologic Stage of CaP Based on Clinical Stage (TNM), PSA, and Gleason Score

Clinical Stage T1c (nonpalpable, PSA elevated) N = 4419

PSA Range (ng/mL)	Pathologic Stage	Biopsy Gleason Score			
		5–6	3 + 4 = 7	4 + 3 = 7	8–10
0–2.5	Organ confined (N = 226)	93 (91–95)	82 (76–87)	73 (64–80)	77 (65–85)
	Extraprostatic extension (N = 19)	6 (5–8)	14 (10–18)	20 (14–28)	16 (11–24)
	Seminal vesicle (+) (N = 1)	0 (0–1)	2 (0–5)	2 (0–5)	3 (0–8)
	Lymph node (+) (N = 3)	0 (0–1)	2 (0–6)	4 (1–12)	3 (1–12)
2.6–4.0	Organ confined (N = 619)	88 (86–90)	72 (67–76)	61 (54–68)	66 (57–74)
	Extraprostatic extension (N = 92)	11 (10–13)	23 (19–27)	33 (27–39)	26 (19–34)
	Seminal vesicle (+) (N = 8)	1 (0–1)	4 (2–7)	5 (2–8)	7 (3–13)
	Lymph node (+) (N = 1)	0 (0–0)	1 (0–1)	1 (0–3)	1 (0–3)
4.1–6.0	Organ confined (N = 1266)	83 (81–85)	63 (59–67)	51 (45–56)	55 (46–64)
	Extraprostatic extension (N = 297)	16 (14–17)	30 (26–33)	40 (34–45)	32 (25–40)
	Seminal vesicle (+) (N = 37)	1 (1–1)	6 (4–8)	7 (4–10)	10 (6–15)
	Lymph node (+) (N = 12)	0 (0–0)	2 (1–3)	3 (1–6)	3 (1–6)
6.1–10.0	Organ confined (N = 989)	81 (79–83)	59 (54–64)	47 (41–53)	51 (41–59)
	Extraprostatic extension (N = 281)	18 (16–19)	32 (27–36)	42 (36–47)	34 (26–42)
	Seminal vesicle (+) (N = 36)	1 (1–2)	8 (6–11)	8 (5–12)	12 (8–19)
	Lymph node (+) (N = 5)	0 (0–0)	1 (1–3)	3 (1–5)	3 (1–5)
>10.0	Organ confined (N = 324)	70 (66–74)	42 (37–48)	30 (25–36)	34 (26–42)
	Extraprostatic extension (N = 165)	27 (23–30)	40 (35–45)	48 (40–55)	39 (31–48)
	Seminal vesicle (+) (N = 25)	2 (2–3)	12 (8–16)	11 (7–17)	17 (10–25)
	Lymph node (+) (N = 13)	1 (0–1)	6 (3–9)	10 (5–17)	9 (4–17)

(continued)

Table 5 Nomograms Predicting Pathologic Stage of CaP Based on Clinical Stage (TNM), PSA, and Gleason Score (*Continued*)

Clinical Stage T2a (palpable < $\frac{1}{2}$ of one lobe) N = 998

PSA Range (ng/mL)	Pathologic Stage	Biopsy Gleason Score			
		5–6	3 + 4 = 7	4 + 3 = 7	8–10
0–2.5	Organ confined (N = 156)	88 (84–90)	70 (63–77)	58 (48–67)	63 (51–74)
	Extraprostatic extension (N = 18)	12 (9–15)	24 (18–30)	32 (24–41)	26 (18–36)
	Seminal vesicle (+) (N = 2)	0 (0–1)	2 (0–6)	3 (0–7)	4 (0–10)
	Lymph node (+) (N = 1)	0 (0–1)	3 (1–9)	7 (1–17)	6 (1–16)
2.6–4.0	Organ confined (N = 124)	79 (75–82)	57 (51–63)	45 (38–52)	50 (40–59)
	Extraprostatic extension (N = 49)	20 (17–24)	37 (31–42)	48 (40–55)	40 (30–50)
	Seminal vesicle (+) (N = 5)	1 (0–1)	5 (3–9)	5 (3–10)	8 (4–15)
	Lymph node (+) (N = 0)	0 (0–0)	1 (0–2)	2 (0–5)	2 (0–4)
4.1–6.0	Organ confined (N = 171)	71 (67–75)	47 (41–52)	34 (28–41)	39 (31–48)
	Extraprostatic extension (N = 101)	27 (23–31)	44 (39–49)	54 (47–60)	46 (37–54)
	Seminal vesicle (+) (N = 10)	1 (1–2)	7 (4–10)	7 (4–11)	11 (6–17)
	Lymph node (+) (N = 3)	0 (0–1)	2 (1–4)	5 (2–8)	4 (2–9)
6.1–10.0	Organ confined (N = 142)	68 (64–72)	43 (38–48)	31 (26–37)	36 (27–44)
	Extraprostatic extension (N = 99)	29 (26–33)	46 (41–51)	56 (49–62)	47 (37–56)
	Seminal vesicle (+) (N = 12)	2 (1–3)	9 (6–13)	9 (5–14)	13 (8–20)
	Lymph node (+) (N = 6)	0 (1–0)	2 (1–4)	4 (2–8)	4 (1–8)
>10.0	Organ confined (N = 36)	54 (49–60)	28 (23–33)	18 (14–23)	21 (15–28)
	Extraprostatic extension (N = 47)	41 (35–46)	52 (46–59)	57 (48–66)	49 (39–59)
	Seminal vesicle (+) (N = 9)	3 (2–5)	12 (7–18)	11 (6–17)	17 (9–25)
	Lymph node (+) (N = 7)	1 (0–3)	7 (3–14)	13 (6–24)	12 (5–22)

Table 5 Nomograms Predicting Pathologic Stage of CaP Based on Clinical Stage (TNM), PSA, and Gleason Score (*Continued*)

Clinical Stage T2b (palpable > $\frac{1}{2}$ of lobe) or T2c (palpable both lobes) N = 313

PSA Range (ng/mL)	Pathologic Stage	Biopsy Gleason Score			
		5–6	3 + 4 = 7	4 + 3 = 7	8–10
0–2.5	Organ confined N = 16	84 (78–89)	59 (47–70)	44 (31–58)	49 (32–65)
	Extraprostatic extension (N = 10)	14 (9–19)	24 (16–33)	29 (19–42)	24 (14–36)
	Seminal vesicle (+) (N = 0)	1 (0–3)	6 (0–14)	6 (014)	8 (0–21)
	Lymph node (+) (N = 0)	1 (0–3)	10 (2–25)	19 (4–40)	17 (3–42)
2.6–4.0	Organ confined (N = 28)	74 (68–80)	47 (39–56)	36 (27–45)	39 (28–50)
	Extraprostatic extension (N = 15)	23 (18–29)	37 (28–45)	46 (36–55)	37 (27–48)
	Seminal vesicle (+) (N = 3)	2 (1–5)	13 (7–21)	13 (7–22)	19 (9–32)
	Lymph node (+) (N = 2)	0 (0–1)	3 (0–7)	5 (0–14)	4 (0–13)
4.1–6.0	Organ confined (N = 46)	66 (59–72)	36 (29–43)	25 (19–32)	27 (19–37)
	Extraprostatic extension (M = 40)	30 (24–36)	41 (33–47)	47 (38–55)	38 (28–48)
	Seminal vesicle (+) (N = 7)	4 (2–6)	16 (10–23)	15 (9–23)	22 (13–33)
	Lymph node (+) (N = 4)	1 (0–2)	7 (3–12)	13 (6–21)	11 (4–23)
6.1–10.0	Organ confined (N = 53)	62 (55–68)	32 (26–38)	22 (17–29)	24 (17–33)
	Extraprostatic extension (N = 28)	32 (26–38)	41 (33–49)	47 (38–56)	38 (29–48)
	Seminal vesicle (+) (N = 15)	5 (3–8)	20 (13–28)	19 (11–28)	27 (16–39)
	Lymph node (+) (N = 5)	1 (0–2)	6 (3–11)	11 (5–19)	10 (3–20)
>10.0	Organ confined (N = 8)	46 (39–53)	18 (13–24)	11 (7–15)	12 (7–18)
	Extraprostatic extension (N = 15)	41 (34–50)	40 (31–51)	40 (30–52)	33 (22–46)
	Seminal vesicle (+) (N = 10)	7 (4–12)	23 (15–33)	19 (10–29)	28 (16–42)
	Lymph node (+) (N = 8)	5 (2–8)	18 (9–30)	29 (15–44)	26 (12–44)

Makarov DV, Trock BJ, Humphreys EB, Mangold LA, Walsh PC, Epstein JI, Partin AW. Updated nomogram to predict pathologic stage of prostate cancer given prostate-specific antigen level, clinical stage, and biopsy gleason score (partin tables) based on cases from 2000 to 2005. *Urology* 2007; 69: 1095–1101.

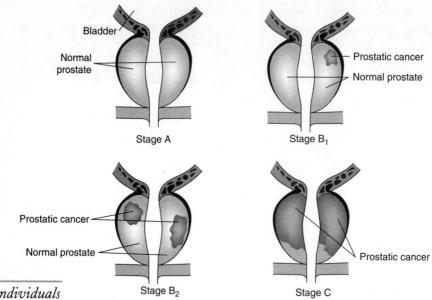

Figure 8   The prostate gland showing the different stages of cancer.

Bone scan

A specialized nuclear medicine study that allows one to detect changes in the bone that may be related to metastatic prostate cancer.

prostate and lymph nodes). Another staging system is the Whitmore Jewett System (**Table 6**).

In individuals in whom there is a concern about metastases to the bone, such as those with high PSAs and pain localized to a bone, a bone scan may be obtained to determined if there are bone metastases.

A **bone scan** is a study performed in the nuclear medicine department that involves injecting a small amount of a radioactive chemical through a vein into your bloodstream. The chemical circulates through your body and is picked up by areas of fast bone growth that may be associated with cancer. The bone scan is the most sensitive technique currently available for identifying prostate cancer that has spread to the bones. Other problems of

Prostate Cancer

Table 6 Prostate Cancer Staging Systems

TNM	Description	Whitmore-Jewett	Description
TX	Primary tumor cannot be assessed	None*	None
T0	No evidence of primary tumor	None	None
T1	Clinically unapparent tumor—not palpable or visible by imaging	A	Same as TNM
T1a	Tumor found incidentally in tissue removed at TUR; 5% or less of tissue is cancerous	A1	Same as TNM
T1b	Tumor found incidentally at TUR; more than 5% of tissue is cancerous	A2	Same as TNM
T1c	Tumor identified by prostate needle biopsy because of PSA elevation	None	None
T2	Palpable tumor confined within the prostate	B	Same as TNM
T2a	Tumor involves half of a lobe or less	B1N	Tumor involves half of a lobe or less; surrounded by normal tissue
T2b	Tumor involves more than half of a lobe, but not both lobes	B1	Tumor involves less than one lobe
T2c	Tumor involves both lobes	B2	Tumor involves one entire lobe or more
T3	Palpable tumor extending through prostate capsule and/or involving seminal vesicle(s)	C1	Tumor < 6 cm in diameter
T3a	Unilateral extracapsular extension	C1	Same as TNM

(Continued)

35

Table 6 **Prostate Cancer Staging Systems** *(Continued)*

TNM	Description	Whitmore-Jewett	Description
T3b	Bilateral extracapsular extension	C1	Same as TNM
T3c	Tumor invades seminal vesicle(s)	C1	Same as TNM
T4	Tumor is fixed or invades adjacent structures other than seminal vesicles	C2	Tumor <6 cm in diameter
T4a	Tumor invades bladder neck and/or external sphincter and/or rectum	C2	Same as TNM
T4b	Tumor invades levator muscle and/or is fixed to pelvic wall	C2	Same as TNM
N+	Involvement of regional lymph nodes	D1	Same as TNM
None	None	D0	Elevation of prostatic acid phosphatase only (enzymatic assay)
NX	Regional lymph nodes cannot be assessed	None	None
N0	No regional lymph node metastasis	None	None
N1	Metastasis in a single regional lymph node, ≤ 2 cm in greatest dimension	D1	Same as TNM
N2	Metastasis in a single regional lymph node, > 2 cm but not > 5 cm in greatest dimension, or multiple regional lymph nodes, none > 5 cm in greatest dimension	D1	Same as TNM
N3	Metastasis in a regional lymph node > 5 cm in greatest dimension	D1	Same as TNM
M+	Distant metastatic spread	D2	Same as TNM

Table 6 Prostate Cancer Staging Systems (*Continued*)

TNM	Description	Whitmore-Jewett	Description
MX	Presence of distant metastases cannot be assessed	None	None
M0	No distant metastases	None	None
M1	Distant metastases	D2	Same as TNM
M1a	Involvement of nonregional lymph nodes	D2	Same as TNM
M1b	Involvement of bone(s)	D2	Same as TNM
M1c	Involvement of other distant sites	D2	Same as TNM
None	None	D3	Hormone refractory disease

*None, No comparable category; TUR, Transurethral resection; PSA, prostate-specific antigen.

Source: Loughlin, P. *100 Questions and Answers About Prostate Disease.* Jones and Bartlett Publishers, LLC, 2007.

Problems of the bones, such as a history of a broken bone, arthritis, and Paget's disease, may cause an increase in uptake of the radioactive chemical.

Osteoblastic lesion

Pertaining to plain X-ray of a bone, increased density of bone seen on X-ray when there is extensive new bone formation due to cancerous destruction of the bone.

Osteolytic lesion

Pertaining to plain X-ray of a bone, refers to decreased density of bone seen on X-ray when there is destruction and loss of bone by cancer.

Hydronephrosis

Dilation of the kidneys, usually due to obstruction.

the bones, such as a history of a broken bone, arthritis, and Paget's disease, may cause an increase in uptake of the radioactive chemical. Often, your history, the location of the bone, and possible additional studies, such as a plain X-ray study or an MRI, will help determine whether the area of increased uptake indicates the presence of cancer.

The bone scan is quite sensitive, but it does not identify small numbers of cancer cells in the bones. In a small number of men (8%), the bone scan may be normal when bone metastases are present. Prostate cancer is not the only cancer that spreads to the bone, but prostate cancer tends to cause the bone to look different than that of involvement with other cancers, such as breast, colon, and bladder. Prostate cancer metastases are typically osteoblastic, whereas those of other cancers tend to be osteolytic. **Osteoblastic lesions** look as if there is an increase in the amount of bone present on a plain X-ray, whereas **osteolytic lesions** look like there is a loss of bone. The bone scan may also show obstruction of the urinary tract, leading to **hydronephrosis**.

The bone scan is often obtained as part of the staging work-up in men with prostate cancer and is helpful in men with a rising PSA (either after primary treatment, such as radical prostatectomy, or during watchful waiting) with or without bone pain to identify new areas of uptake that may indicate new bone involvement. The bone scan is usually obtained as part of the staging evaluation in men with newly diagnosed clinically localized prostate cancer who have a PSA > 20 ng/mL. Because the risk of bone metastases in men with newly diagnosed clinically localized prostate cancer who have a PSA ≤ 20 ng/mL is so low, a bone scan is not routinely obtained in these men. Although the chemical used for the study is radioactive, the amount used is small, and it will not put you or your family at-risk.

17. What is a pelvic lymph node dissection and what are the risks?

If it goes outside of the prostate, the first location to which prostate cancer tends to spread is the pelvic lymph nodes. It is important to know whether the cancer has spread to the lymph nodes because the success rates of treatments such as interstitial seed therapy and radical prostatectomy are lower if the cancer has spread into the pelvic lymph nodes. Thus, the urologist or radiation oncologist should have a good idea whether there is prostate cancer involvement of the pelvic lymph nodes before recommending a therapy. Unfortunately, radiologic studies such as CT scans have not been helpful in identifying individuals with smaller amounts of cancer in the pelvic lymph nodes. CT or MRI may be warranted for staging men with high-risk clinically localized prostate cancer and PSA values > 20.0 ng/ml or when the Gleason score is greater than or equal to 8.

The most accurate way to assess the lymph node status is to remove the lymph nodes and have them examined by the pathologist. The lymph nodes to which prostate cancer typically spreads are located in the lateral aspect of each side of the pelvis (see Question 12). Removing the lymph nodes requires surgery, either an open procedure or a laparoscopic procedure, and has risks. The use of the ProstaScint scan to detect prostate cancer in the pelvic lymph nodes is being evaluated.

Not everyone needs a pelvic lymph node dissection. When the risk of having positive lymph nodes is low, such as occurs in men with a low Gleason score and a PSA < 10 ng/ml, a lymph node dissection is unnecessary, and one can proceed directly with definitive therapy, such as interstitial seed therapy, external beam radiation therapy (EBRT), and radical prostatectomy. In high-risk patients, those with higher Gleason scores (8–10), or those with a PSA > 10 ng/ml, a lymph node dissection may be performed at the same time as a planned radical prostatectomy, before planned EBRT, or before interstitial seed therapy. If an open prostatectomy or laparoscopic robotic prostatectomy is planned, the lymph nodes can be removed using the same approach as for the prostatectomy and can be examined by the pathologist (frozen section) just before the prostatectomy. Frozen section specimens are interpreted by the pathologist shortly after they are removed from the patient, and the findings are reported to the surgeon in the operating room. The surgeon then decides whether to proceed with removal of the prostate based on whether cancer has been identified in the lymph nodes. Some surgeons remove the prostate in the presence of small amounts of cancer in the lymph nodes, whereas others do not. The slides are then made into permanent sections and reviewed again by the pathologist. In most cases, the interpretation of the frozen section is the same as that of the permanent section; rarely do the two differ. In a perineal prostatectomy, the perineal incision does not allow access to the pelvic lymph nodes, and a separate midline incision or a laparoscopic approach is needed for the lymph node dissection. With EBRT or interstitial seed therapy, the pelvic lymph node dissection may be performed laparoscopically or via an open incision that is located below the umbilicus on a separate day, before EBRT/interstitial seeds.

A lymph node dissection should be performed in high-risk patients because it may affect treatment. The likelihood of having positive nodes varies with the stage of the prostate cancer, the PSA value, and the Gleason score. Approximately 5–12% of men who are believed to have clinically localized prostate cancer (low stage) have cancer that has spread to the pelvic lymph nodes. Before the pelvic lymph node dissection, you should discuss with your doctor how your planned prostate cancer treatment would be affected if you had cancer involving the pelvic lymph nodes.

The main risks of a pelvic lymph node dissection are bleeding, nerve injury, and lymphocele. The obturator nerve supplies muscles in the leg and is surrounded by some of the pelvic lymph nodes. If this nerve is damaged at the time of surgery and not repaired, it may lead to permanent inability to cross your leg on the side of the injury. A lymphocele is a collection of lymph fluid that accumulates in the pelvis, resulting from injury the lymph vessels. Lymphoceles require treatment if they are large and causing pressure/pain and/or become infected. Usually they can be drained by placing a small drainage tube through the skin into the lymphocele.

Before the pelvic lymph node dissection, you should discuss with your doctor how your planned prostate cancer treatment would be affected if you had cancer involving the pelvic lymph nodes.

18. What options do I have for treatment of my prostate cancer?

Cliff's comment:

After finally realizing that, despite feeling great, I did indeed have prostate cancer, I had to figure out what the best treatment for me was. When faced with the option of leaving my prostate in place or removing it, I knew that, even though I was petrified of surgery, it would be the best thing for me in the long run. I knew that I could not live with my prostate gland and the continuous question of whether there were any viable cancer cells remaining in my prostate after interstitial seeds or radiation therapy.

Various treatment options are available for prostate cancer, each with its own risks and benefits (**Table 7**). The options available may vary with the grade of tumor, the extent of tumor spread, your overall medical health and life expectancy and your personal preferences. The treatments for prostate cancer can be divided into those that are intended to "cure" your cancer (definitive therapies) and those that are **palliative**, intended to slow down the growth of the prostate cancer and treat its symptoms. Definitive therapies for localized prostate cancer include: interstitial seed therapy (brachytherapy), external beam radiation (EBRT), and radical prostatectomy (open, laparoscopic, or robotic). Other therapies, such as cryotherapy, high intensity focused ultrasound (HIFU), and combination therapy (external beam radiation plus interstitial seed therapy) are not commonly used for men with localized prostate cancer.

Palliative therapies for prostate cancer include the use of hormonal therapies and radiation therapy for symptomatic bone metastases. In those individuals whose prostate cancer is refractory to hormonal therapy, chemotherapy may be an option.

The option of **watchful waiting** and **active surveillance** can also be chosen. Watchful waiting involves no treatment initially. Rather, your prostate cancer is monitored with periodic PSAs and DREs and possibly X-rays. The premise of watchful waiting is that some individuals will not benefit from definitive treatment for their prostate cancer. With watchful waiting, palliative treatment (treatment designed to slow down the growth of the

Palliative

Treatment designed to relieve a particular problem without necessarily solving it. For example, palliative therapy is given in order to relieve symptoms and improve quality of life, but it does not cure the patient.

Watchful waiting

Active observation and regular monitoring of a patient without actual treatment.

Active surveillance

An alternative to immediate treatment for men with presumed low-risk prostate cancer. Involves close monitoring and withholding active treatment unless there is a significant change in the patient's symptoms or PSA.

Table 7 Treatment Options for Prostate Cancer

Mode of Treatment	Advantages	Disadvantages	Curative: Yes/No	Alternative If Fails
Hormonal therapy • Therapy in which the male hormones (androgens) are eliminated from the body. • Primary treatment for older men with prostate cancer who don't want surgery or forms of XRT but also don't want to watch and wait. • Also used as therapy for men with metastatic disease.	1. Orchiectomy: A one time procedure that avoids the need for shots; it drops testosterone quickly to almost zero and is permanent. 2. LHRH analogues and antagonists: Not permanent.	1. Orchiectomy: Permanent outpatient procedure involves minor surgery, risk of infection, bleeding, pain. 2. LHRH: Can have flair of bone pain in those with bone metastases; need to pretreat these men with androgen receptor blocker; requires monthly to yearly visits/or shots, which can be expensive. Antagonists don't cause flair. 3. Antiandrogen therapy: Blocks cells' ability to absorb the hormone often used in conjunction with shots. Most antiandrogens are not effective as a single agent, however. Diarrhea, liver damage, impaired night vision. 4. Casodex monotherapy: Gynecomastia. Not approved in the U.S. Not permanent.	No: Hormone therapy stops the growth of those prostate cancer cells that are hormone sensitive. Used for treatment of metastatic diagnosis.	Chemotherapy

(Continued)

Table 7 Treatment Options for Prostate Cancer (*Continued*)

Mode of Treatment	Advantages	Disadvantages	Curative: Yes/No	Alternative If Fails
Cryotherapy	Minimally invasive, no blood loss. Quicker recovery; one-time procedure; can be used in those who cannot undergo RRPX or as salvage procedure for local recurrence after XRT.	Impotence, urethral strictures, urinary retention, urinary frequency, dysuria, hematuria, penile or scrotal swelling, fistula, incomplete treatment of cancer. Works better on smaller prostates; more difficult to perform if prior TURP (transurethral resection of prostate); incontinence up to 30% when used as salvage procedure.	Used primarily for XRT failures, but can be used as first line therapy.	Hormone treatment, radical prostatectomy, but there is increased risk of complication.
External beam radiation therapy	One-time procedure that may cure prostate cancer in earlier stages. Allows for pathologic staging of disease. PSA goes to undetectable if no remaining prostate cancer.	Incontinence; impotence; bladder neck contracture. Rarely: a need for blood transfusion, nerve injury, rectal injury. Longer recovery period, 2–4% incidence of permanent incontinence. 20–40% incidence of permanent impotence.	Yes, in setting of localized diagnosis.	If it fails locally, external beam radiation therapy is used. If it fails in distant disease (metastases), hormones are used.

Prostate Cancer

Table 7   Treatment Options for Prostate Cancer (Continued)

Mode of Treatment	Advantages	Disadvantages	Curative: Yes/No	Alternative If Fails
External beam radiation therapy	Avoids major surgery; may cure prostate cancer in early stages. Incontinence and impotence less common than with surgery. No transfusion risk.	Fatigue; skin reaction in treated areas; urinary frequency and dysuria; proctitis, rectal bleeding, frequent stools, urgency; bowel function may remain abnormal; hematuria. Rare: fistula. No lymph node analysis or pathologic staging; requires treatments 5 days a week for 6 to 7 weeks; 30–50% chance of erectile dysfunction; 10–15% chance of bladder and/or rectal irritation. May have hair loss in area receiving full dose such as pubic hair. PSA doesn't go to undetectable levels.	Yes, in setting of localized diagnosis.	Hormone treatment, which is palliative. Salvage prostatectomy with associated increased risk of incontinence.
Laparoscopic radical prostatectomy & robotic-assisted radical prostatectomy	Quicker recovery; less postoperative pain; possible better visualization of pelvic anatomy. Allows for accurate staging; same advantages as RRPX. Less blood loss compared to open radical prostatectomy. Robotic vs. lap—faster OR time, easier to perform. Comparable short-term outcomes to open surgery.	Laparoscopic A long procedure that was first pioneered by French in 1998; long-term data not available. Steep learning curve. Robot is extremely expensive.	Yes, if localized diagnosis.	Locally, XRT; in distant disease, hormones are used.

45

Table 7 Treatment Options for Prostate Cancer (*Continued*)

Mode of Treatment	Advantages	Disadvantages	Curative: Yes/No	Alternative If Fails
Brachytherapy (interstitial seeds)	Minimally invasive; quick recovery, short hospitalization; no transfusions.	This therapy is not for every patient (men with high grade cancer, PSA > 10, Gleason score ≥ 7, are more likely to fail). Large glands are more difficult. Urinary frequency, urgency, hematuria, rectal irritation, pain, burning, frequency and urgency with bowel movements. Chance of impotence or pain with ejaculation; 25–60% chance of impotence. No pathologic staging; urinary retention; harder to do if have had prior TURP.	Over the short term, if the diagnosis is localized, brachytherapy appears to be curative; long-term data need to be reviewed.	Salvage prostatectomy if localized; hormones if distant disease.
Chemotherapy	1. Kills and/or reduces growth of cancer. 2. Provides palliation (symptom relief).	Potentially significant side effects.	Some chemotherapy combinations have been shown to improve outcomes and significantly prolong survival.	

cancer and to treat symptoms, but not cure the cancer) is instituted for local or metastatic progression, if it occurs. Palliative therapies include: trimming of the prostate (transurethral prostatectomy) if the prostate becomes large enough that it causes trouble urinating, hormonal therapy to decrease the size and growth of the prostate cancer and radiation therapy if symptomatic bone metastases occur.

Active surveillance differs from watchful waiting. The goal of active surveillance is to give definitive treatment to those men with prostate cancers that are likely to progress and to decrease the risk of treatment related side effects in those men whose cancers are less likely to progress. Thus, with active surveillance one also undergoes periodic PSAs and DREs, but definitive therapy is instituted when predefined changes are noted. There are no established active surveillance protocols, although studies are ongoing. You and your doctor would need to discuss a mutually agreeable protocol before starting active surveillance.

Monitoring with active surveillance is often more frequent than with watchful waiting. Active surveillance is better for older patients with shorter life expectancies and with lower risk prostate cancers

Surgery is currently the most commonly performed treatment with the intent to cure prostate cancer. The surgical procedure is called a radical prostatectomy (see Question 20) and involves the removal of the entire prostate gland. Radical prostatectomy may be performed through an **incision** that extends from the umbilicus to the pubic bone (**Figure 9**), through a perineal incision (between the scrotum and the anus) (**Figure 10**), laparoscopically (**Figure 11**), and more recently with the

Surgery is currently the most commonly performed treatment with the intent to cure prostate cancer.

Incision

Cutting of the skin at the beginning of surgery.

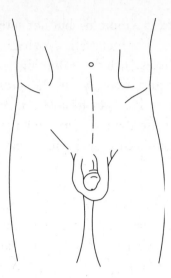

Figure 9   Surgical incisions for radical retropublic prostatectomy. A midline incision is made from the symphysis pubis to the umbilicis.

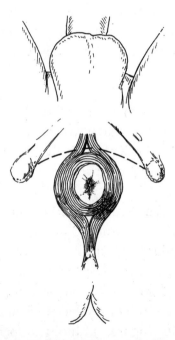

Figure 10   Radial perinal prostatectomy—incision lines.

Reprinted with permission from Gibbons RP, Radical Perineal Prostalectomy. Definitive Treatment for Patients with Localized Prostate Cancer. AUA Update Series, Vol. 13, Lesson 5. AUA Office of Education, Houston, TX 1994.

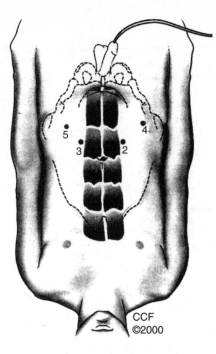

Figure 11   Trocar sites for laparoscopic radial prostalectomy.

Reprinted with permission from *The Urologic Clinics of America,* Volume 28, Number 2, May 2001, p. 424. © WB Saunders Company.

assistance of a robot (**Figure 12**). The choice of technique varies with the patient's body characteristics and the urologist's preference.

Interstitial seed placement (**brachytherapy**) is a procedure that is gaining in popularity because it is minimally invasive and requires a single treatment. Similar to radical prostatectomy, it is a procedure with intent to cure. This procedure involves the **percutaneous** placement of radioactive seeds into the prostate (see Question 22, Figure 13). Depending on the prostate cancer grade and stage and the PSA, conformal external-beam radiation therapy (EBRT), in which beams of

Interstitial

Within an organ, such as interstitial brachytherapy, whereby radioactive seeds are placed into the prostate.

Brachytherapy

A form of radiation therapy whereby radioactive pellets are placed into the prostate.

Percutaneous

Through the skin.

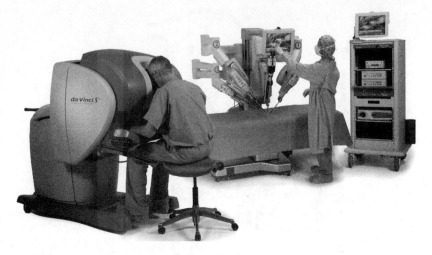

Figure 12   The da Vinci surgical system.

© 2009 Intuitive Surgical, Inc. Used with Permission.

high-energy radiation are aimed at the prostate (or other target organ), may be used in addition to the interstitial seeds.

Conformal EBRT

EBRT that uses CT scan images to better visualize radiation targets and normal tissues.

Conformal EBRT is a newer way of delivering EBRT to the prostate (see Question 23). Through the use of CT scanning and the improved ability to focus the maximum radiation effects on the prostate and less on the surrounding tissues, conformal EBRT may decrease side effects and improve results over those of traditional EBRT. This procedure is also performed with intent to cure.

Cryotherapy

A prostate cancer therapy in which the prostate is frozen to destroy the cancer cells.

Cryotherapy is a minimally invasive procedure in which probes are percutaneously placed into the prostate under ultrasound guidance. Liquid nitrogen is administered through the probes to freeze and kill the cancer cells (see Question 25). Currently, this procedure is more commonly used as a second-line procedure when an individual has not responded to EBRT. However, it, too, is used with intent to cure.

High-intensity focused ultrasound (HIFU) is a procedure that is being performed in Europe and appears to be an option for lower Gleason score prostate cancers and for local recurrence of prostate cancer after external beam radiation therapy. The procedure is performed by inserting a probe into the rectum. The probe delivers highly focused ultrasound to the prostate. The high intensity focused ultrasound heats the prostate to temperatures of 80–100 degrees centigrade, which is enough to kill prostate cancer cells. The effect is limited to the prostate and does not irritate the rectal tissue. HIFU is not currently approved for use in the United States.

Hormone therapy, through the use of pills, shots, both pills and shots, or bilateral orchiectomy, is a palliative approach to the treatment of prostate cancer. By removing or preventing the action of testosterone on the prostate cancer, these therapies shrink the prostate cancer and slow down its growth. However, they do not cure prostate cancer (see Question 26).

Hormone therapy

The manipulation of the disease's natural history and symptoms through the use of hormones.

Various chemotherapy regimens are being evaluated to identify drugs that may be effective against prostate cancer. The ideal drug would be one that kills the prostate cancer, rather than just slowing down its growth. Recently, the Food and Drug Administration has approved the use of certain chemotherapies for men with hormone resistant prostate cancer (see Question 28). Clinical trials are being performed to identify new medications and combinations of medications in hopes of identifying more effective therapies with fewer side effects. You can contact your nearby medical center to see if they are participating in any clinical trials for prostate cancer.

Radiation therapy

Use of radioactive beams or implants to kill cancer cells.

Radiation therapy is typically used as palliative treatment for patients with pain caused by bone metastases.

Intravenous (IV) medications, such as pamidronate, may also be used to treat painful bone metastases, and suramin may also be helpful in patients with extensive bone metastases (see Question 30).

Chemotherapy

A treatment for cancer that uses powerful medications to weaken and destroy the cancer cells.

Chemotherapy is the use of powerful drugs either to kill cancer cells or to interfere with their growth. Chemotherapy drugs are good at fighting cancer because they affect mostly fast-multiplying cancer cells. Some healthy cells in the body also divide quickly, such as cells that produce hair, blood, nails, and the lining of the mouth and intestinal tract. Cells in these parts of the body can be harmed by chemotherapy. Therefore, some common side effects of chemotherapy include hair loss, low white blood cell count, nail changes, mouth and throat irritation, nausea, and vomiting.

Chemotherapy can be either injected into a vein or taken by mouth. The medicine then travels throughout the body to reach some cancer cells that may have spread beyond the prostate. Often, patients who are given hormone therapy prior to chemotherapy continue their hormone treatment through the course of their chemotherapy. In studies, this treatment offered no survival benefit and helped only to reduce pain (see Question 28).

19. How do I decide which treatment is best for me?

Currently, the burden of medical decision making falls on you, the patient, and it is our job as physicians to provide you with the information that will allow you to make the decision. When forced to make a difficult decision, we often rely on loved ones, close friends, and knowledgeable individuals to help us, but these people do not have to live with the effects of that decision. As you weigh the pros and cons of each of the various treatment options, it is very important that you think of how they will affect you. Now is the time to be very honest with yourself about what side effects you can and cannot tolerate. It is your physician's responsibility to accurately inform you of the likelihood of side effects of each of the treatment options and the remedies that are available to treat those side effects. When faced with a diagnosis of prostate cancer, the first impulse may be to get rid of the cancer at any cost. Unfortunately, once the prostate cancer has been treated and that worry quiets down, the side effects of the treatment can become more bothersome—so you should think seriously about them beforehand.

When counseling a patient, the first question that I typically ask is "Can you live with your prostate inside of you over the long term?" If the answer is no, that you would be constantly worrying about whether cancer remained in the prostate if it were left in place, then a radical prostatectomy is probably best for you. Other issues to bear in mind are the impact of incontinence and erectile dysfunction on your lifestyle. Virtually all forms of therapy can cause erectile dysfunction. If this is particularly worrisome to you, then it may be appropriate to meet with an urologist who treats erectile dysfunction to discuss the treatment options before you begin treatment for your prostate cancer. Similarly, it may be helpful to discuss the various treatments for incontinence or inability to urinate (**retention**) with your urologist or radiation oncologist before undergoing treatment. Your physician may make some treatment recommendations based on your age, medical conditions, and

Retention

Difficulty in emptying the bladder of urine; may be complete, in which one is unable to void, or partial, in which urine is left in the bladder after voiding.

clinical stage of your prostate cancer. If you have questions as to why certain recommendations are being made, now is the time to ask them. Remember, no question is stupid. Your physician wants you to feel comfortable with your decision and will help you find the information that you need. There are also organizations that can provide you with information regarding treatment and side effects (see Appendix B).

In an effort to help determine which therapies have the best chance of curing you of your prostate cancer, researchers have stratified prostate cancer into low-risk, intermediate-risk, and high-risk for disease progression. The treatment recommendations vary with the risk.

Low-risk:

T1c or T2a prostate -cancer

PSA < 10 ng/mL

Gleason score ≤ 6

Intermediate-risk:

Clinical stage T2b

Gleason score 7

PSA 10 ng/mL–20 ng/mL

High-risk:

Clinical stage T2c or higher

PSA > 20 ng/ml

Gleason score 8–10

Low-risk patients usually do well with a single therapy, such as radical prostatectomy, external beam radiation therapy, or interstitial seed therapy. High-risk patients are more likely to experience a treatment failure, and combination therapy, such as external beam therapy and hormonal therapy, is often recommended.

20. What is a radical prostatectomy? Are there different types?

Cliff's comment:

It has been 10 years since my radical prostatectomy, and I feel great. I am doing all of the things that I had done before the surgery and more. So far, my PSA has remained undetectable, and it is very reassuring to hear this at my urology clinic visits.

Radical prostatectomy is the surgical procedure whereby the entire prostate is removed, as well as the seminal vesicles, the section of the urethra that passes through the prostate, the ends of the vas deferens, and a portion of the bladder neck. After the prostate and surrounding structures are removed, the bladder is then reattached to the remaining urethra. A **catheter**, which is a hollow tube, is placed through the penis into the bladder before the stitches that attach the bladder to the urethra are tied down. The catheter allows urine to drain while the bladder and urethra heal together. In open radical prostatectomy a small drain is often placed through the skin of the abdomen into the pelvis. This drain allows for drainage of lymph and urine that may occur during the first few days after the surgery. This drain is removed when the fluid output decreases. At the time of radical prostatectomy, depending on the approach used, the pelvic lymph nodes, which are a common location of prostate cancer metastases, may also be removed (see

Radical prostatectomy is the surgical procedure whereby the entire prostate is removed, as well as the seminal vesicles, the section of the urethra that passes through the prostate, the ends of the vas deferens, and a portion of the bladder neck.

Catheter

A hollow tube that allows for fluid drainage from or injection into an area.

Question 12). A radical prostatectomy may be performed via three different approaches. A common form is the open retropubic approach, in which an incision is made that extends from the umbilicus (belly button) to the symphysis pubis (pubic bone) (Figure 9). The radical prostatectomy may also be performed laparoscopically through several small incisions made in various locations in the abdomen (Figure 11), or through a perineal approach, with the incision being made in the area between the scrotum and the anus (Figure 10). More recently, the radical prostatectomy may be performed with the use of a robot, robotic-assisted radical prostatectomy, which has quickly become the most popular technique for radical prostatectomy.

Radical prostatectomy differs from a transurethral resection of the prostate (TURP) and an open suprapubic prostatectomy in that the entire prostate is removed in a radical prostatectomy. Therefore, unlike TURP and open suprapubic prostatectomy, the PSA should decrease to an undetectable level within a month or so after the procedure if no prostate cancer cells are present.

The decision as to what approach will be used for a radical prostatectomy depends on your urologist's preference and skills, your body characteristics, and whether a pelvic lymph node dissection is planned.

An advantage of the retropubic approach is that it allows for easy access to the pelvic lymph nodes so that a pelvic lymph node dissection can be performed easily at the same time. In addition, the blood vessels and nerves that control your potency are visualized easily. A disadvantage of this procedure is the abdominal incision, which may lead to a longer recovery time and increased discomfort and a higher blood loss compared to laparoscopic and robotic-assisted radical prostatectomy.

The **perineal prostatectomy** does not involve an abdominal incision, is reported to be less uncomfortable and the recovery period shorter. The perineal approach allows for good visualization of the outlet of the bladder and the urethra for sewing the two together; however, the nerves that control potency are not seen as easily as with the retropubic approach. Another disadvantage of this procedure is that it does not allow for removal of the pelvic lymph nodes through the perineal incision and would require an additional incision for the pelvic lymph node dissection. This procedure is best suited for overweight men, for whom the retropubic approach is more difficult.

Laparoscopic radical prostatectomy is a procedure that has the advantages of the retropubic approach but, because there are several small abdominal incisions as opposed to the longer midline incision, the discomfort is less and the recovery is quicker with this approach. The disadvantage of this procedure is that it is relatively new and requires a urologist with advanced skills in **laparoscopy**. It may take longer to perform than an open radical retropubic prostatectomy. The outcomes of laparoscopic prostatectomy, such as urinary incontinence, erectile function, and **positive margin** rates are similar to open surgery. Robotic-assisted radical prostatectomy has surpassed laparoscopic radical prostatectomy in terms of the number of procedures being performed.

Robotic-assisted prostatectomy is the newest form of minimally invasive surgery for prostate cancer. The procedure is performed using a three-armed robot. The robot is controlled by the surgeon, who sits at a specialized desk and controls movement of the robot's arms. Advantages of robotic-assisted prostatectomy are its ease of use compared to laparoscopy and the surgery

Perineal prostatectomy

Removal of the entire prostate, seminal vesicles, and part of the vas deferens through an incision made in the perineum.

Laparoscopic radical prostatectomy

Removal of the entire prostate, seminal vesicles, and part of the vas deferens via the laparoscope.

The perineal prostatectomy does not involve an abdominal incision, is reported to be less uncomfortable and the recovery period shorter.

Laparoscopy

Surgery performed through small incisions with visualization provided by a small fiberoptic instrument and fine instruments that fit through the small incisions.

Positive margin

The presence of cancer cells at the cut edge of tissue removed during surgery. A positive margin indicates that there may be cancer cells remaining in the body.

Robotic-assisted radical prostatectomy

A radical prostatectomy performed with the assistance of a robot.

Laparoscopic

Performed with a laparoscope.

Nerve-sparing prostatectomy

Form of radical prostatectomy whereby an attempt is made to spare the nerves involved in erectile function.

Dissect

The surgical removal of tissue.

tends to be quicker as compared to laparoscopy. In addition, the arms of the robot have movements similar to a human arm/hand/wrist, but the tremors that may be present with human movements are controlled. A disadvantage of the robot is the expense of the robot, so not all hospitals can afford to purchase one. The outcomes with the robot are similar to those of **laparoscopic** and open radical prostatectomy; however, long-term outcomes are limited for the robot and are limited for laparoscopy (Figure 12).

What is a nerve-sparing radical prostatectomy?

The nerves responsible for erectile function run along each side of the prostate and along each side of the urethra before passing out of the pelvis into the penis. These nerves travel along with blood vessels, and the group is called the *neurovascular bundle*, which lies outside of the prostate capsule. These nerves are not responsible for control of urine, only erectile function. During a **nerve-sparing prostatectomy**, the urologist attempts to **dissect** the neurovascular bundle from the prostate and the urethra. The surgeon may perform a bilateral nerve-sparing radical prostatectomy, in which the neurovascular bundle on each side is spared, or a unilateral nerve-sparing prostatectomy, in which one neurovascular bundle is removed with the prostate. The decision of whether or not to perform a nerve-sparing radical prostatectomy depends on many issues, one of which is your erectile function. If you already have erectile dysfunction, then sparing the nerves is not an issue. Other considerations include the amount of tumor present in your biopsy specimen, the location of the tumor (whether it is in both sides of the prostate), and the Gleason score. Remember that a radical prostatectomy is a cancer operation, and the goal of the procedure is to try to remove all of the cancer. Therefore, if you are at high risk for having cancer at the edge of the prostate, it is better to remove the neurovascular bundle(s) and surrounding tissue on that side in hopes of removing all of the cancer. A bilateral nerve-sparing radical prostatectomy does not guarantee that you will have normal erectile function after the surgery. You should consider this fact and decide before surgery how much of an impact postoperative erectile dysfunction would have on your life.

What is the success rate of radical prostatectomy?

In general, more than 70% of properly selected patients (i.e., men who are believed to have prostate cancer that is clinically confined to the prostate) remain free of tumor for more than 7 to 10 years. If one has a T2 tumor, the probability of remaining free from PSA elevation can be as high as 90% if there were no positive margins. However, it is hard to predict before surgery who is the best candidate for surgery because 30 to 40% of patients are diagnosed with a higher stage or grade of cancer when the surgical specimen is reviewed by the pathologist. Positive surgical margins are found in 14 to 41% of men undergoing radical prostatectomy, and in those men with positive margins, there is an almost 50% chance that the PSA will increase within 5 years after surgery. This varies with the amount of tumor at the margin and the location of the positive margin. Your urologist would discuss whether additional therapy is indicated if the margin is positive. Men with negative margins have only an 18% chance of the PSA rising at 5 years after surgery. Initially after surgery, you will have your PSA level checked every 3 months. Depending on the lab that your physician uses, a PSA level < 0.1 ng/mL or a PSA level < .02 ng/mL may be reported as undetectable. The numbers vary because the **sensitivity** in PSA testing varies from lab to lab. If the PSA remains undetectable after 1 year, then your urologist may order PSA testing every 6 months for about 1 year, after

Sensitivity

The probability that a diagnostic test can correctly identify the presence of a particular disease.

which you will continue with yearly PSA tests. Depending on your pathology report and your urologist's preference, you may also have a digital rectal examination at the time of your PSA.

Cliff's comment:

The first PSA test after surgery is the most suspenseful. Even though your urologist may tell you that your pathology specimen from surgery looks good and that there are no cancer cells at the the edges of the tissue, you are still anxious to hear what the PSA is. You want it to be undetectable—want it to indicate that the cancer has been caught and removed. You get your blood drawn and then you wait to meet with your urologist or for the phone call regarding your results. I remember how happy I felt when I got my first PSA report after the surgery. Now, $2^{1}/_{2}$ years later, I am still slightly anxious when I have my PSA drawn, although as each year goes by the anxiety is decreasing. With each good PSA result, I start to believe that they've gotten it all. I can technically say that I am cured, but each year that goes by that I am healthy and the PSA remains undetectable is another year enjoyed and another closer to that goal.

Who is a candidate for radical prostatectomy?

The ideal candidate for a radical prostatectomy is a man who is believed to have prostate cancer that is confined to the prostate gland, is healthy enough to withstand the general anesthesia and the surgical procedure, and is expected to live for at least an additional 7 to 10 years so that he will benefit from the surgery. It is difficult to determine who really has organ-confined disease, which is cancer that is apparently confined to the prostate. Tables may help estimate the risks of having tumor outside of the prostate, but these are only part of the decision making process. Approximately 20 to 60% of men undergoing radical prostatectomy have a higher stage of prostate cancer when the pathologist reviews the surgical specimen.

Just because you are a candidate for a radical prostatectomy does not mean that this is the best form of treatment for you. You must look carefully at your lifestyle, the risks of the surgery, and what is most important to you regarding your quality of life before making a decision. If, for example, the possibility of urinary incontinence would be devastating to you, then maybe surgery is not the best therapy for you. On the other hand, if the idea of leaving your prostate in place will constantly worry you, then perhaps surgery is best for you.

21. What are the risks of surgery? How are they treated?

All surgical procedures have risks, and the common ones are infection, bleeding, pain, and anesthetic complications. Larger surgical procedures, which involve lengthier operative times and decreased postoperative mobility, have the risk of blood clots in the legs (deep venous thrombosis), pulmonary embolus, pneumonia, and stress-related stomach ulcers. Complications of radical prostatectomy include **hernia**, significant bleeding requiring blood transfusion, infection, anesthetic-related complications, impotence, urinary incontinence, bladder neck contracture, deep venous thrombosis, rectal injury, and death.

Hernia

A weakening in the muscle that leads to a bulge, often in the groin.

Bleeding

In most cases, the blood loss is less than one pint (**unit**) of blood, but in about 5 to 10% of cases, a blood transfusion is required. The amount of blood loss tends to be lower with both laparoscopic and robotic-assisted radical

Unit

Term referring to a pint of blood.

prostatectomies, compared to open radical retropubic prostatectomy.

Infection

Several different types of infections can occur with this surgery. A skin infection (cellulitis) may occur at the incision, an abscess may occur under the skin or deep in the pelvis, or a urinary tract infection may occur. A skin infection at the incision typically presents with redness, swelling, tenderness, and occasionally, drainage at the incision. In the absence of pus, this usually can be treated successfully with oral antibiotics; rarely, intravenous antibiotics are indicated.

Abscesses are collections of pus and may occur just under the skin or deeper in the pelvis and require drainage. More superficial abscesses can be treated by opening the incision, draining the pus, and packing the wound with sterile gauze. The packing is continued until the area heals. If the abscess is in the pelvis, it can often be treated by placing a drain through the skin into the abscess and draining the pus. This is often done under X-ray guidance by an interventional radiologist.

Urinary tract infections result from the catheter, which drains the bladder during the healing process. The risk of a urinary tract infection increases with the number of days that the catheter is in place. Because most urologists leave the catheter in for 1 to 2 weeks after the surgery, your urologist may have you drop a urine sample off at the lab 2 to 3 days before the catheter is removed so that they can detect whether any bacteria is present and if so, treat the bacteria to prevent an infection after the catheter has been removed. Signs of a urinary tract infection include frequent urination, urgency and discomfort with urination, and sometimes a low-grade fever.

Anesthetic Complications

Most patients undergo **general anesthesia** for their radical prostatectomy; however, the procedure may be performed under spinal anesthesia. **Epidural anesthesia** may be used frequently to improve postoperative pain control and decrease intraoperative anesthetic requirements. The most commonly encountered side effects of general anesthesia are scratchy throat, nausea, and vomiting, but significant anesthetic complications are rare. With epidural catheters, potential side effects include lowering of the blood pressure and muscle blocks, which may affect movement of a leg.

Impotence

Impotence, or **erectile dysfunction**, is unfortunately a commonly identified risk of radical prostatectomy. The nerves that supply the penis and that are involved in the erectile process lie along each side of the prostate and the urethra. They may be taken deliberately by the surgeon (non-nerve-sparing radical prostatectomy), or they may be injured permanently or transiently. The decision to try to spare one or both nerve bundles varies with your surgeon's expertise, your Gleason score, your PSA level, and the volume of tumor on the biopsies. The incidence of postoperative erectile dysfunction may be as low as 25% in men younger than 60 years who undergo bilateral nerve-sparing radical prostatectomy, or it may be as high as 62% in men older than 70 years who undergo unilateral nerve-sparing radical prostatectomy. Many factors can affect your erectile function after surgery, including your erectile function before surgery, your age, your pathological tumor stage, and the extent of preservation of the nerves. Erectile dysfunction after radical prostatectomy may resolve over the first year or two after surgery. During that time and if the trouble persists, you may seek treatment for it (see Part Three section on erectile

Prostate Cancer

General anesthesia
Anesthesia which involves total loss of consciousness.

Epidural anesthesia
A special type of anesthesia whereby pain medications are placed through a catheter in the back, into the fluid that surrounds the spinal cord.

Erectile dysfunction
The inability to achieve and/or maintain an erection satisfactory for the completion of sexual performance.

dysfunction). After a radical prostatectomy, you have no ejaculate because the sources of the fluid are either removed (prostate and seminal vesicles) or tied off (the vas deferens). However, you should still experience climax (reach an orgasm).

Urinary Incontinence

Urinary incontinence is another risk of radical prostatectomy. Incontinence may vary from none to persistent incontinence, such that every time you move you leak urine. The more common type of incontinence is stress-related incontinence, leakage that occurs when you increase the pressure in your abdomen, such as when you bear down, pick up something heavy, laugh, or cough. The incidence of incontinence varies from 1 to 58%, and one of the reasons for the wide range in the reported incidence of incontinence is that the definition of incontinence varies. If one considers any leakage to be incontinence, then the incidence would be higher than if incontinence were defined as leakage sufficient to change a pad a day. As with erectile dysfunction, incontinence may improve or resolve over time. Risks for incontinence after surgery include prior pelvic irradiation and older age. Many options are available for the treatment of urinary incontinence after radical prostatectomy (see Question 24).

Cliff's comment:

I feared this risk the most. I remember getting the diapers and pads the day I had my catheter removed. "My God," I thought, "I am 60 years old and I'm going to be wearing diapers." Needless to say, my wife has no sympathy when I moaned about the possibility of having to wear a pad. I was lucky, however; I had two small "spills" at night and that was it for my incontinence. I discarded all of those diapers and pads within a week.

Bladder Neck Contracture

A **bladder neck contracture** is scar tissue that develops in the area where the bladder and urethra are sewn together. This problem occurs in about 1 in every 20 to 30 prostatectomies. The signs and symptoms of a bladder neck contracture include decreased force of stream and straining (pushing) to urinate. The bladder neck contracture is identified during an office cystoscopy, in which a **cystoscope**, a telescope-like instrument, is passed through the urethra up to the bladder neck and the narrowed area is visualized. If the opening is very small, a small wire can be passed through it and the area dilated using some metal or plastic dilators. Before the procedure, the urethra is numbed with lidocaine jelly to decrease discomfort. Usually, once the bladder neck is dilated, it remains open; however, in a small number of men, a repeat dilation or an incision into the scar under anesthesia is needed. A complication of treatment for bladder neck contracture is urinary incontinence.

Deep Venous Thrombosis

A **deep venous thrombosis (DVT)** is a blood clot that develops in the veins in the leg or the pelvis. People with cancer and those who are sedentary are at increased risk for such blood clots. Thromboembolic (TED) hose and Venodynes (pneumatic sequential stockings that inflate and deflate to keep blood flowing) are often used during surgery and the postoperative period to decrease the risk of forming such blood clots. DVTs may cause swelling of the leg, which often resolves when the blood clot dissolves. A more serious risk posed by a DVT is that a piece of the clot could break off and travel to the heart and lungs. This is called a pulmonary embolus. A pulmonary embolus can be life threatening if the fragment is large enough to block off blood flow to the lung.

Bladder neck contracture

Scar tissue at the bladder neck that causes narrowing.

Cystoscope

A telescope-like instrument that allows one to examine the urethra and inside of the bladder.

Deep venous thrombosis (DVT)

The formation of a blood clot in the large deep veins, usually of the legs or in the pelvis.

Prostate Cancer

Rectal Injury

The incidence of rectal injury during a radical prostatectomy is less than 2%. There is a slightly higher risk of rectal injury with the perineal approach (1.73%) than with the retropubic approach (0.68%). In most cases, if the injury is small and you have performed the bowel prep and no stool is visible, then the area can be closed and should heal. For large injuries that occur with bowels that are not well prepped, a temporary **colostomy** is made to decrease the chances of stool leakage and abscess formation; the colostomy can be taken down later.

Miscellaneous Complications Related to the Radical Prostatectomy

The retropubic prostatectomy has a higher risk of cardiovascular, respiratory, and other medically related complications, primarily **gastrointestinal**, such as slow return of bowel function, than the perineal approach. The perineal approach has a higher risk of miscellaneous surgical complications, such as rectal injury and postoperative infections. The perineal approach may also be associated with an increased risk of incontinence of stool. The incidence of complications and **mortality** increases with patient age at the time of surgery.

Death

The mortality rate associated with radical prostatectomy is less than 0.1%.

22. What is brachytherapy/interstitial seed therapy? Who is a candidate? What are the risks?

Brachytherapy derives from the Greek word *brachy*, which means *near to*. Brachytherapy is a technique in which either permanent radioactive seeds (**Figure 13**) or

Colostomy

A surgical opening between the colon (large intestine) and the skin that allows stool to drain into a collecting bag.

Gastrointestinal (GI)

Related to the digestive system and/or the intestines.

Mortality

Death related to disease or treatment.

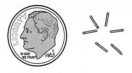

Figure 13   Actual size of I-125 seeds used for brachytherapy.

temporary needles are placed directly into the prostate gland. Palladium 103 and iodine 125 are two radioactive agents that can be used for permanent seed placement and both are effective in the treatment of prostate cancer. Palladium gives a higher initial dose of radiation when it is placed, and some people think that it may be more helpful in high-grade, fast-growing tumors. Palladium tends to be used for tumors with a Gleason score of at least 7, and iodine is used for tumors with a Gleason score of 6 or lower. Before the seeds are placed, either a transrectal ultrasound or a CT scan of the prostate is performed to assess the prostate volume. This helps determine needle placement and seed positioning within the needle. Typically, the target volume includes the original prostate volume plus 2-mm margins laterally and anterior to the prostate gland, as well as additional 5-mm margins at the top and bottom of the prostate. This measurement is done to try to ensure that the prostatic capsule is included in the treatment. No additional margins are added posteriorly to prevent injury to the rectum. It is also important to limit the dose received by the urethra to prevent urethral irritation. Typically, a dose of 144 Gy is given for iodine 125, and 125 Gy is given for palladium 103. Iodine 125 has a half-life of 60 days, whereas palladium has a half-life of only 17 days.

The most commonly encountered side effects of interstitial seed therapy include voiding troubles related to bladder outlet obstruction, urinary incontinence, and rectal ulceration and bleeding. In addition, in some patients a benign increase in the PSA may occur after interstitial seed therapy. Urinary symptoms occur earlier with palladium because it releases high energy earlier than iodine. Individuals may develop urinary **frequency**, dysuria, or urinary retention. Urinary symptoms, if they are not associated with urinary retention, are often treated with nonsteroidal anti-inflammatories and an alpha-blocker, such as doxazosin (Cardura), terazosin (Hytrin), alfuzosin (Uroxatral), tamsulosin (Flomax) and silodosin (Rapaflo). They often resolve over 1 to 4 months, but may persist for 12 to 18 months.

Bladder Outlet Obstruction

Trouble urinating after interstitial seed therapy occurs in 7 to 25% of patients, possibly as a result of blood clots in the bladder or swelling of the prostate. About 10% of men will experience **acute urinary retention** requiring temporary placement of a Foley catheter. Your doctor may want you to try some medications, including an alpha-blocker, such as doxasin (Cardura), terazosin (Hytrin), tamsulosin (Flomax) or silodosin (Rapaflo), and/or an anti-inflammatory (e.g., ibuprofen) (see Question 39). If you are not able to void for awhile, then a suprapubic tube or clean intermittent **catheterization** may be easier for you. A suprapubic tube is a catheter that is placed through the skin of the lower abdomen into the bladder to drain the urine. It remains in place until you can urinate on your own. It has the advantages of being able to be changed on a monthly basis in your urologist's office, and it does not cause urethral irritation like a Foley catheter.

Clean intermittent catheterization involves placing a catheter through the penis into the bladder to drain the

---

Frequency

A term used to describe the need to urinate 8 or more times per day.

Acute urinary retention

The inability to pass urine from the bladder.

Catheterization

The passage of a catheter into the bladder to empty the bladder of urine.

Clean intermittent catheterization

The placement of a catheter into the bladder to drain urine and the removal after the urine is drained at defined intervals throughout the day, to allow for bladder emptying. It may also be performed to maintain patency after treatment of a bladder neck contracture or urethral stricture.

bladder on a regular schedule (usually every 4 to 6 hours) throughout the day. The advantages of clean intermittent catheterization are that it allows you to know when you are able to void on your own, it minimizes bladder and urethral irritation, and it has less risk of infections and bladder stones over the long term. Although it is discouraging to be unable to urinate after the procedure, it is important to allow time to pass and see whether the problem will resolve. A TURP should be delayed to give you a sufficient trial because of the increased risk of urinary incontinence.

Urinary Incontinence

Urinary incontinence is uncommon in men undergoing interstitial seed therapy affecting < 1%. However, in men who have had a prior TURP, the risk of incontinence is 25% and is up to 40% if more than one TURP has been performed.

Rectal Ulceration/Bleeding

Rectal irritation does not occur as commonly as urinary symptoms and tends to improve quicker than urinary symptoms do. Fewer than 5% of patients will have a rectal ulcer or rectal bleeding, which occurs as a result of irritation of the rectal lining. It may be associated with pain, rectal spasms, and the feeling that one needs to have a bowel movement. This condition can be treated with several topical medications, including Anusol, hydrocortisone, Proctofoam hydrocortisone, mesalamine (Rowasa) suppositories, Metamucil, and a low-roughage diet.

PSA "Bounce" or "Blip"

This occurs when the PSA increases on two consecutive blood draws and then decreases and remains low without rising again. The cause of this phenomenon is not

Clean intermittent catheterization involves placing a catheter through the penis into the bladder to drain the bladder on a regular schedule (usually every 4 to 6 hours) throughout the day.

known. It occurs in about one-third of men treated with interstitial seeds and typically occurs around 9 to 24 months after the treatment. It may or may not be accompanied by symptoms of prostate inflammation; if such symptoms are present, then treatment for prostatitis may decrease the symptoms and the PSA level.

Urethral Stricture

This narrowing of the urethra is related to the development of scar tissue and occurs in 5 to 12% of men, and tends to develop later. It may present with a change in the force of stream or the need to strain to void. A stricture is identified by cystoscopy in the doctor's office. Treatment of the stricture depends on the location and the extent of the stricture; it may require simple office dilation or an incision under anesthesia.

Erectile Dysfunction

This condition may occur in as many as 40 to 60% of men who undergo interstitial seed therapy. Unlike radical prostatectomy, the erectile dysfunction tends to occur a year or more after the procedure and not right away. As with post radical prostatectomy ED, there are a variety of options available to treat it (see Part Three, Erectile Dysfunction).

Who is a candidate for interstitial seed therapy?

Similar to radical prostatectomy, the goal of interstitial therapy is to cure the patient of prostate cancer. With this in mind, the candidate should have a life expectancy of more than 7 to 10 years and no underlying illness that would contraindicate the procedure such that he will not benefit from a cure. Men with significant obstructive voiding symptoms and/or prostate volumes greater than 60 mL are at increased risk for voiding troubles and urinary retention after the procedure. Men who have undergone a prior TURP are at increased risk for urinary incontinence after brachytherapy. Men with clinically localized prostate cancer of low to intermediate risk are candidates for interstitial seed therapy. Men with high-risk prostate cancer (PSA > 20 ng/mL, Gleason score > 8, or stage T3a prostate cancer) should not be treated with interstitial seed therapy alone. Depending on your risk, hormonal therapy may be used in addition to interstitial seed therapy.

Men with clinically localized prostate cancer of low to intermediate risk are candidates for interstitial seed therapy.

In some individuals who are deemed to be at higher risk, external beam radiation therapy may be used in addition to interstitial seed therapy. Interstitial seed therapy is limited in its ability to reach tissue outside of the prostate, especially the back of the prostate. The addition of EBRT may help in patients who are judged to be at high risk for disease penetrating through or outside the prostate capsule. Use of interstitial seeds alone is appropriate for patients with tumors in clinical stage T1c to T2a, a Gleason score < 6, and a PSA < 10. Patients with a Gleason score of 7 or greater, a PSA > 10, tumors in clinical stage T2b or minimal T3a, and at least four of six biopsies positive for cancer or perineural invasion on the biopsy appear to be the best served by the combination of interstitial seeds and EBRT.

How is one monitored after interstitial seed therapy and what is the success rate?

Unlike with radical prostatectomy, the prostate remains in your body, and thus the PSA does not decrease to an undetectable level. In addition, it may take at least 2 years for the PSA to reach its lowest level (**PSA nadir**). The PSA is typically checked 1 month after seed

PSA nadir

The lowest value that the PSA reaches during a particular treatment.

placement, then every 3 to 6 months for 2 years thereafter if the level remains stable. After 2 years, the PSA is checked yearly. In January 2005 the definition of PSA failure after radiation therapy was refined. The Phoenix definition defines PSA failure after radiation therapy as a rise by 2 ng/ml or more above the nadir PSA with or without the use of androgen blockade.

A rise in PSA may occur in as many as one third of the patients between the first and second year after the implantation. This is called a *benign PSA bump*, and it appears to be related to late tissue reactions to the radiation, but it does not mean that the seeds have failed or that you are at increased risk of failure. In this situation, the PSA does not continue to rise, and this is how one differentiates a PSA bump from a failure.

The results of prostate brachytherapy are comparable to those of radical prostatectomy for 5 to 7 years after treatment. The long-term data (i.e., the data for longer than 10 years after treatment) are limited. Reported studies demonstrate success rates of 64 to 85% at ten years, with success being defined by either a PSA < 0.5 ng/mL or the absence of three consecutive rises in PSA in patients who received brachytherapy EBRT.

23. What are external-beam and conformal external-beam radiation therapies? What are the side effects of EBRT?

External-beam radiation therapy (EBRT) is the use of radiation therapy to kill or inactivate cancer cells. The total radiation dose is given in separate individual treatments, known as *fractionation*. Cancer cells are most sensitive to radiation at different phases in their growth.

By giving the radiation on a daily basis, the radiation oncologist hopes to catch the cancer cells in the sensitive phases of growth and also to prevent the cells from having time to recover from the radiation damage. Conformal EBRT uses CT images to help better visualize the radiation targets and the normal tissues. With three dimensional images, the radiation oncologist can identify critical structures, such as the bladder, the rectum, and the hip bones. This allows the radiation oncologist to deliver more radiation (72–82 Gy as opposed to 66–72 Gy with standard EBRT) to the prostate tissue but decrease the amount of normal tissue that is irradiated. The advantage of conformal EBRT over EBRT is that conformal EBRT causes less rectal and urinary irritation. The construction of an immobilization device (cradle) and the placement of small, permanent tattoos ensure that you are properly positioned for the radiation treatment each day. Through the assistance of computers, the radiation oncologist can define an acceptable dose distribution to the prostate and surrounding tissues, and the computer determines the appropriate beam configuration to create this desired distribution.

By giving the radiation on a daily basis, the radiation oncologist hopes to catch the cancer cells in the sensitive phases of growth and also to prevent the cells from having time to recover from the radiation damage.

Who is a candidate for conformal EBRT?

Men who are candidates for conventional EBRT are also candidates for conformal EBRT. Similar to other curative treatments, the ideal patient has a life expectancy of 7 to 10 years. In higher-risk patients, the increased radiation dose used with conformal EBRT causes a significantly better decrease in PSA progression than the dose used in conventional EBRT. There does not appear to be a PSA progression-free survival benefit with conformal EBRT when compared with conventional EBRT in patients who have low-risk prostate cancer. Men who have a PSA level > 10 ng/mL or with a tumor that is

Prostate Cancer

clinical stage T3 are the most likely to benefit from the higher radiation doses that can be achieved with conformal EBRT. They may benefit from combination therapy, such as hormone therapy for 6 months plus EBRT. For patients with locally advanced or high-grade disease (Gleason score > 7) studies have demonstrated that 2 to 3 years of postradiation adjuvant therapy helps improve survival. The amount of radiation and the field of radiation differ for each individual and depend on the clinical stage and the Gleason grade. Contraindications to EBRT include a history of inflammatory bowel disease, such as Crohn's disease and ulcerative colitis or a history of prior pelvic radiotherapy.

What are the side effects and risks of EBRT and conformal EBRT?

The side effects of EBRT or conformal EBRT can be either acute (occurring within 90 days after EBRT) or late (occurring > 90 days after EBRT). The severity of the side effects varies with the total and the daily radiation dose, the type of treatment, the site of treatment, and the individual's tolerance. The most commonly noted side effects include changes in bowel habits, bowel bleeding, skin irritation, edema, fatigue, and urinary symptoms, including dysuria, frequency, hesitancy, and nocturia. Less commonly, swelling of the legs, scrotum, or penis may occur. Late side effects include persistence of bowel dysfunction, persistence of urinary symptoms, urinary bleeding, urethral stricture, and erectile dysfunction.

Bowel Changes

A change in bowel habits is one of the more common side effects of EBRT. Patients may develop diarrhea, abdominal cramping, the feeling of needing to have a bowel movement, rectal pain, and bleeding. Usually, if these side effects are going to occur, they do so in the second or third week of treatment.

Rectal pain can be treated with warm sitz baths, hydro-cortisone-containing creams (ProctoFoam HC, Corti-foam), or anti-inflammatory suppositories (Anu-sol, Rowasa).

Late bowel effects include persistent changes in bowel function, rectal **fistula**, or perforation (a hole in the rec-tum), and bleeding. Rectal fistula and perforation are rare and often require surgical treatment.

Skin Irritation

How skin tolerates radiation depends on the dose of radiation used and the location of the skin affected. The perineum and the fold under the buttocks are very sen-sitive and may become red, flake, or drain fluid. To pre-vent further irritation, avoid applying soaps, deodorants, perfumes, powders, cosmetics, or lotions to the irritated skin. After you wash the area, gently blot it dry. Cotton underwear and loose fitting clothes can help prevent further irritation. If the irritated skin is dry, topical ther-apies, such as petroleum jelly (Vaseline), lanolin, zinc oxide, Desitin, Aquaphor, Procto-Foam, and corn starch, can be applied.

Edema

Edema of the legs, scrotum, and penis may rarely occur, but when it does, it is more common in those who have undergone prior pelvic lymph node dissection. Lower extremity edema can be treated with supportive stock-ings, TED hose, and elevation of feet when sitting and lying down. Penile and scrotal edema is often difficult to treat.

Fistula

An abnormal passage or communication, usually between two internal organs, or leading from an internal organ to the surface of the body.

How skin tolerates radiation depends on the dose of radiation used and the location of the skin affected.

Urinary Symptoms

The genitourinary symptoms of dysuria, frequency, hesitancy, and nocturia are related to changes that occur in the bladder and urethra that result from radiation exposure. The bladder may not hold much urine because of the irritation and scarring, and irritation of the bladder lining may make it more prone to bleeding. Bladder inflammation usually occurs about 3 to 5 weeks into the radiation treatments and gradually subsides about 2 to 8 weeks after the completion of radiation treatments. Urinary anesthetics (phenazopyridine HCL [Pyridium]) and bladder relaxants (antimuscarinic agents) may be helpful in decreasing the urinary frequency.

What is the success rate with EBRT/conformal EBRT?

The success rate varies with the initial PSA level. In one study, 89 to 92% of men treated with conformal EBRT whose pretreatment PSA was < 10 ng/mL showed no increase in PSA level at 5 years. Those with a pretreatment PSA of 10 to 19.9 ng/mL had an 82 to 86% chance of no increase in PSA level at 5 years, compared with a 26 to 63% chance of no increase in PSA at 5 years in men with a pretreatment PSA of > 20 ng/mL.

Men with T1 and T2 tumors have survival rates that are comparable to that with radical prostatectomy. In such individuals, the clinical tumor-free survival is 96% at 5 years and 86% at 10 years.

24. What if I am incontinent after radical prostatectomy or radiation therapy? What if I have erectile dysfunction after radical prostatectomy or EBRT or brachytherapy?

When seeking treatment for prostate cancer, many men are very concerned about the effects of the treatment on erectile function. Basically, all of the treatment options carry a risk of erectile dysfunction; however, they differ in how soon after treatment the erectile dysfunction occurs and how likely it is to occur. If you are already having trouble with erections, none of the treatments for prostate cancer will improve your erections. The incidence of erectile dysfunction associated with radical prostatectomy varies with patient age, erectile function before surgery, nerve-sparing status, and the surgeon's technical ability to perform a nerve-sparing radical prostatectomy. The incidence of erectile dysfunction after a nerve-sparing radical prostatectomy varies from 16 to 82%. When it occurs with radical prostatectomy, erectile dysfunction is immediate and is related to damage of the pelvic nerves, which travel along the outside edge of the prostate. Men who have undergone nerve-sparing radical prostatectomies and who are impotent after surgery may experience return of their erectile function over the following 12 months.

The incidence of erectile dysfunction after EBRT ranges from 32 to 67% and is caused by radiation-related damage to the arteries. Unlike with surgery, the erectile dysfunction occurs a year or more after the radiation. The incidence of erectile dysfunction is 15 to 31% in the first year after EBRT and 40 to 62% at 5 years after EBRT.

The incidence of erectile dysfunction after interstitial seed therapy with or without medium-dose EBRT ranges from 6 to 50%. Similar to EBRT, the erectile dysfunction tends to occur later than with radical prostatectomy.

Hormone therapy with the LHRH analogues or orchiectomy also causes erectile dysfunction, as well as loss of interest in sex in most men. This loss of libido is related to the loss of testosterone, but why the loss of testosterone causes troubles with erections is not well known.

Various therapies are available for the treatment of erectile dysfunction, including oral, intraurethral, and injection therapies; the vacuum device; and the **penile prosthesis**, which is a device that is surgically placed into the penis and allows an impotent individual to have an erection (see Questions 75, 80–100).

Penile prosthesis

A device that is surgically placed into the penis that allows a man with erectile dysfunction to have an erection.

In the treatment of post-radical prostatectomy erectile dysfunction, the effectiveness of oral PDE-5 Inhibitors (Viagra, Cialis, Levitra) varies with nerve-sparing status:

Bilateral nerve sparing: 71% success rate

Unilateral nerve sparing: 50% success rate

Non–nerve sparing: 15% success rate

In men with EBRT-associated erectile dysfunction, oral PDE-5 Inhibitors work in about 70% of individuals. In men who have erectile dysfunction associated with interstitial seed therapy, PDE-5 Inhibitors have a success rate of approximately 80% (see Question 81 for use of PDE-5 inhibitors).

If oral therapy is not effective or if you have contraindications to oral therapy there are a variety of other medications/devices that may allow you to achieve an adequate erection for satisfactory sexual function. See Questions 84–99.

Urinary incontinence, the uncontrolled loss of urine, is one of the most bothersome risks of prostate cancer treatment. Although it is more commonly associated with radical prostatectomy, it may also occur after interstitial seed therapy, EBRT, and cryotherapy. Urinary incontinence may lead to anxiety, hopelessness, and loss of self-control and self-esteem. Fear of leakage may limit social activities and participation in sex. If you are experiencing these feelings, you should discuss this with your doctor and spouse or significant other.

If you experience persistent urinary incontinence after surgery or radiation therapy, your doctor will want to identify the degree and the type of incontinence. You will be asked questions regarding the number of pads you use per day, what activities precipitate the incontinence, how frequently you urinate, if you have frequency or urgency, how strong your force of urine stream is, if you feel that you are emptying your bladder well, and what types and how much fluid you are drinking. The doctor may check to make sure that you are emptying your bladder well. This is usually done by having you urinate and then scanning your bladder with a small ultrasound probe to determine how much urine is left behind. Normally, less than 30 cc (one tablespoon) remains after urination.

Several different types of urinary incontinence exist, and the different types may coexist. The treatment of urinary incontinence varies with the type, and the types that may be encountered in men being treated for prostate cancer includes stress, overflow, and urge incontinence. Men who have undergone radical prostatectomy typically experience a type of stress incontinence called *intrinsic sphincter deficiency*. Stress incontinence may also occur after interstitial seed therapy and is much more common if a TURP of the prostate was performed in the past. In men, urinary control is primarily at the bladder outlet by the internal sphincter muscle. This muscle remains closed and opens only during urination. An additional muscle, the external sphincter, is located further away from the bladder and is the back up muscle. The external sphincter is the muscle that you contract when you feel the urge to urinate and there is no bathroom in sight. During a radical prostatectomy, the internal sphincter is often damaged with removal of the prostate because it lies just at the top of the prostate. Continence then depends on the ability of the remaining urethra to close (**coapt**) and on the external sphincter.

Urge incontinence is the involuntary loss of urine associated with the urge to urinate and is related to an overactive bladder. Although less common than intrinsic sphincter deficiency in men who have undergone radical prostatectomy, it may be present alone or in conjunction with intrinsic sphincter deficiency. Overactive bladder and decreased bladder capacity are more common in men who have undergone EBRT for prostate cancer. Urge incontinence can be treated with antimuscarinic agents, medications which relax the bladder muscle.

Urge incontinence

Incontinence associated with urgency.

Overflow incontinence is the involuntary loss of urine related to incomplete emptying of the bladder. After radical prostatectomy, this may occur if significant scarring (a bladder neck contracture) is present at the bladder outlet area. Treatment of the bladder neck contracture often relieves the overflow incontinence. Other symptoms include a weak urine stream and the feeling of incomplete bladder emptying. With overflow incontinence, the bladder scanner would demonstrate a large amount of urine left in the bladder after urinating. Urethral strictures after EBRT may also cause overflow incontinence; dilation of such strictures also improves

Overflow incontinence

A condition in which the bladder retains urine after voiding, and as a result, urine leaks out, similar to a full cup under the faucet.

the overflow incontinence. Urethral strictures tend to recur, and daily in and out passage of a catheter beyond the site of the stricture helps prevent recurrence of the stricture. Swelling of the prostate after interstitial seed therapy may cause voiding troubles, which if unrecognized, may lead to overflow incontinence. Initial treatment of overflow incontinence after seed therapy is with clean intermittent catheterization, and possibly the addition of an alpha-blocker (Hytrin, Cardura, Flomax, Rapaflo) and a nonsteroidal anti-inflammatory.

Your doctor may wish to perform further studies (see urodynamics in Question 34) to further identify the cause of your incontinence.

Treatment Options

Once the cause and the severity of the urinary incontinence has been assessed, you can then embark on treatment. In all cases of incontinence, it is important to make sure that you are voiding regularly, that is, every 3 hours, and avoiding alcohol and caffeinated fluids. Caffeine and alcohol cause the kidneys to make more urine and are bladder irritants. It may also be helpful to avoid acidic foods and foods with a lot of hot spices because these may also act as bladder irritants.

If a bladder neck contracture is present, treatment may consist of dilation or incision. There is a risk of stress incontinence after incision of a bladder neck contracture. If overflow incontinence occurs after interstitial seed therapy, your doctor may give you a medication called an alpha-blocker to relax the prostate, an anti-inflammatory drug, and prescribe clean intermittent catheterization until you are voiding on your own. Usually, voiding troubles of this nature after interstitial seed therapy resolve with time, so additional treatment is rarely needed. Your doctor will be quite reluctant to do anything more aggressive for the first 6 months after the placement of the seeds because of the high risk of urinary incontinence with a TURP.

Overactive bladder is treated with medications that relax the bladder muscle, the most common of which are called antimuscarinics, including:

- oxybutynin (Ditropan)
- Ditropan XL
- tolterodine (Detrol)
- Detrol LA
- solifenacin (Vesicare)
- trospium chloride (Sanctura)
- Sanctura XR
- darifenacin (Enablex)
- oxybutynin patch (Oxytrol)
- oxybutynin gel (Gelnique)
- fesoterodine (Toviaz)

More common side effects of these medications include dry mouth, facial flushing, constipation, and, in some patients, blurry vision. Dry mouth and constipation rates are decreased with the long-acting formulations.

A variety of treatment options exist for stress incontinence, including pelvic floor muscle exercises, a penile clamp, collagen injection, an artificial sphincter, and a male urethral sling.

Pelvic floor muscle exercises: Pelvic floor muscle exercises are intended to strengthen these muscles. To identify these muscles, simply try stopping your urine stream while you are urinating. The exercises involve repetitive contracting and relaxing of the pelvic muscles at least 20 times per day every day of the week. Pelvic floor stimulation and biofeedback allow you to identify these muscles better and to monitor the strength of the contractions.

Penile clamp: Several penile clamps are available, and all of them have the same principle, which is to compress the urethra to prevent urinary leakage (**Figure 14**). They should be worn for brief periods of time only and should not be left on all day. If they are left on for long periods of time, they may cause damage to the penile skin and the urethra. The clamp needs to be removed if you need to urinate. The penile clamp should not take the place of pelvic floor muscle exercises; rather, it should be used as a backup measure. For instance, if you are going out to dinner and want to make certain there is no leakage, then you should use the penile clamp.

Collagen injection: Collagen is a chemical that is found throughout your body. The collagen that is being used to treat urinary incontinence is derived from a cow. Because it comes from a source outside of your body,

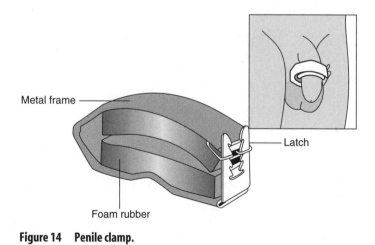

Metal frame

Latch

Foam rubber

Figure 14   Penile clamp.

you must have skin testing to make sure that you are not allergic to the collagen. The collagen is injected into the bladder neck and the proximal urethra to make the ure-thra come together (coapt) (**Figure 15**). The amount of collagen injected at each treatment varies from person to person. The collagen injection can be performed in the urologist's office under local anesthesia or in the operat-ing room under spinal or general anesthesia. More com-monly, the collagen is injected retrograde through a cystoscope that is placed through the penile urethra and positioned just before the injection site. A long, thin needle is then passed through the scope, advanced into the urethra at the appropriate location where the collagen

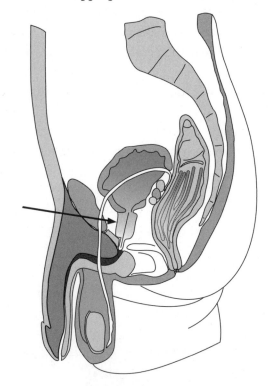

Figure 15   Location of collagen injection.

is injected. The collagen is injected at several sites in the urethra until the urologist is satisfied with the amount of urethral coaptation. Some urologists prefer to perform the procedure antegrade. A small needle is passed through the lower abdominal skin into the bladder. A small wire is then placed through the needle into the bladder, and the needle is removed. Small dilators are then placed over the wire to make an opening that is large enough for the cystoscope, which is then placed through the opening in the abdominal skin into the bladder. The bladder neck is identified and the collagen injected. Often, more than one treatment session is needed. Typically three to four injections, each 4 weeks apart, are necessary. It is also possible that repeat collagen injections will be necessary over the long term. Collagen injections provide a continence rate of about 26% in postprostatectomy incontinence and a reduction in the number of pads used per day in an additional 37% of men.

The advantages of collagen injection are that it is minimally invasive, it is repeatable, it is associated with a short recovery period, and if it fails, it does not prevent you from pursuing other forms of therapy. Disadvantages of collagen therapy are that only a small percentage of men become totally dry, a small number of men develop a urinary tract infection, and 11% of men have transient urinary retention requiring clean intermittent catheterization. Permanent retention has not been reported.

Lastly, some individuals will experience transient dysuria (discomfort with voiding) and urgency after the procedure. The best candidates for collagen are men who have higher Valsalva leak point pressures (60 cm H_2O), who do not have overactive bladders, have not had prior radiation or cryotherapy, and who have not had a vigorous incision of a bladder neck contracture.

Artificial urinary sphincter. The artificial sphincter is a mechanical device that is comprised of a cuff that is placed around the urethra, a pump that is placed in the scrotum, and a reservoir that is positioned in the abdomen (**Figures 16** and **17**). All of these parts and the tubing that connects them are buried under the skin and are not visible. The cuff remains filled with sterile fluid and compresses the urethra. When you wish to urinate, the pump is pressed, which transfers fluid out of the cuff, allowing you to urinate. The cuff automatically refills to compress the urethra. Placement of the artificial sphincter requires general or spinal anesthesia and an overnight hospital stay. Initially after the surgery, the sphincter is

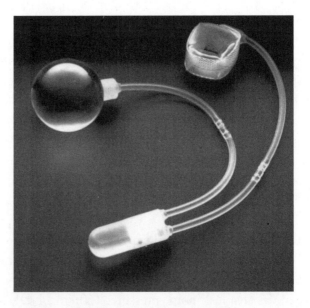

Figure 16   AMS Sphincter 800 urinary prosthesis.

Courtesy of American Medical Systems®, Inc. Minnetonka, Minnesota (www.AmericanMedicalSystems.com).

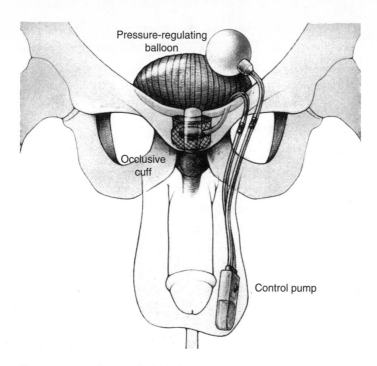

Pressure-regulating balloon

Occlusive cuff

Control pump

Figure 17   Location of artifical sphincter.

Courtesy of American Medical Systems®, Inc. Minnetonka, Minnesota (www.AmericanMedicalSystems.com).

deactivated so that it doesn't work. It will be activated 4 to 6 weeks after surgery, when the tissues have healed and the swelling and sensitivity have subsided. The artificial sphincter provides continence rates of 20 to 90%, including men who are either totally dry or who use one pad per day. The sphincter can be used after collagen has failed. Disadvantages of the sphincter include mechanical malfunction rates of 10 to 15%, erosion rates of 0 to 5%, and infection rates of 3%. The cuff may erode, or move, into the urethra or through the skin, and other parts of the sphincter may erode into the skin or other areas. If there is an erosion, the device must be removed. Similarly, if the sphincter becomes infected, it must be removed. It is very important that a urodynamic study be performed before the sphincter is placed to make sure that the bladder holds an adequate amount of urine at low pressures and to identify an overactive bladder, which would require additional treatment.

Male sling: The fascial sling has been used for several years in women with stress incontinence and has proved to be a successful and durable procedure. Because of its success in women, it has been used more recently in men who are incontinent after radical prostatectomy. The sling may be derived from the patient's own tissues, from a synthetic material, or from cadavers. The goal of the sling is to place tissue under the urethra to act as a buttress or a hammock. The tissue is anchored to either the abdominal wall or the pubic bone.

Success rates with the male sling vary, but about 50% will be dry with a single procedure and retightening of the sling in those who are incontinent after the initial surgery can improve the success rate. In a long-term study, 64% of patients were improved and required two or fewer pads per day after the sling and 36% required zero pads per day. This is a surgical procedure that usually involves an overnight stay in the hospital. Urinary retention may occur that requires CIC over the short term and loosening of the sling if persistent. Complications of surgery include the need for revision, erosion of the sling, and infection.

25. What is cryotherapy/cryosurgery? Who is a candidate? What is the success rate? What are the risks?

Cryotherapy is a technique used for prostate cancer treatment that involves controlled freezing of the prostate gland. First-line cryotherapy treatment is an option, when treatment is appropriate, to men who have clinically organ-confined disease of any Gleason grade with a negative metastatic evaluation. The size of the prostate gland affects the ability to obtain uniform freezing of the prostate and individuals with large prostates may benefit from decreasing the size of the prostate by the use of pretreatment hormone therapy. This procedure is performed under anesthesia. Transrectal ultrasound evaluation, similar to that used with your prostate biopsy, is used throughout the procedure to visualize the prostate and to monitor the position of the freezing probes, which are placed through the perineal skin into the prostate (**Figure 18**). During the freezing, the transrectal ultrasound demonstrates an ice ball in the prostate. The freezing process kills both hormone-sensitive and hormone-insensitive cancer cells. Proper positioning of the probe may allow one to kill cancer cells even at the prostate **capsule**. During the freezing, a catheter is placed into the urethra, and a warming solution is run through the catheter to protect the urethra from freezing.

Capsule

A fibrous outer layer that surrounds the prostate.

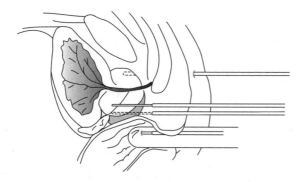

Figure 18   Placement of needles for cryoblation of the prostate.

Who is a candidate for cryotherapy?

Although more commonly used as a **salvage** therapy (a procedure intended to "rescue" a patient after a failed prior therapy) for men who fail to respond to EBRT or interstitial seeds, cryotherapy can be used as a first-line therapy in individuals who have clinically organ-confined disease of any grade with a negative metastatic evaluation. The size of the prostate gland is a factor in patient selection and outcome. The larger the prostate the more difficult it is to achieve a uniformly cold temperature throughout the gland. Thus, those men with large prostate glands may benefit from the addition of hormone therapy (LHRH analogues) to decrease the size of the prostate prior to cryotherapy. A relative contraindication to performing cryotherapy is a large TURP defect. Cryotherapy achieves the best results when the starting PSA is less than 10 ng/ml. Cryotherapy is a minimally invasive option when treatment is appropriate for men who either don't want or who are not good candidates for radical prostatectomy because of comorbidities, including obesity or a history of pelvic surgery. It may also be a reasonable option for men with a narrow pelvis or those who cannot tolerate EBRT, including those with previous nonprostatic pelvic irradiation, inflammatory bowel disease, or rectal disorders. For patients desiring minimally invasive therapy for intermediate disease prostate cancer, Gleason 7 and/or Gleason 8 with PSA > 10 ng/ml and < 20 ng/ml and/or clinical stage T2b, cryotherapy is also an option.

Cryotherapy is a minimally invasive option when treatment is appropriate for men who either don't want or who are not good candidates for radical prostatectomy because of comorbidities, including obesity or a history of pelvic surgery.

What is the success rate of cryotherapy?

In patients who have not responded locally to EBRT, approximately 40% who then undergo salvage cryotherapy have an undetectable PSA level after cryotherapy, and 78% have negative prostate biopsy results. It appears that a drop in the PSA to 0.5 ng/mL after cryotherapy is associated with a good prognosis. In men with post-cryotherapy PSA levels > 0.5 ng/mL, there is a higher likelihood that the PSA will increase or that the prostate biopsy result will be positive. When cryotherapy is used as the initial primary therapy, a PSA lowest value of ≤ 0.5 ng/mL is associated with a better prognosis.

In studies with long-term data ranging from 5–10 years postcryotherapy, the 5-year biochemical disease-free survival rates for low-, intermediate-, and high-risk cases range from 65–92%, 69–89%, and 48–89%, respectively. A multi-center registry (the Cyroablation online database registry) of primary cryotherapy (no prior procedures surgical or radiation-based) reported pooled 5-year biochemical disease-free progression outcomes noting that:

85% of low-risk patients are disease free at 5 years.

73.4% of intermediate-risk patients were disease free at 5 years.

75% of high-risk patients were disease free at 5 years, using the old ASTRO definition of biochemical recurrence/progression which was defined as three consecutive rises in PSA.

Using the "Phoenix biochemical disease free" definition of nadir PSA plus 2 ng/ml, the following results were achieved:

91% biochemical disease-free rate in low-risk patients

78% biochemical disease-free rate in intermediate-risk patients

62% biochemical disease-free rate in high-risk patients

What are the side effects/complications of cryotherapy?

Common side effects of cryotherapy include perineal pain, transient urinary retention, penile and/or scrotal swelling, and hematuria. Urinary retention occurs in roughly 3% of individuals. Anti-inflammatories seem to help, but individuals may require a catheter or suprapubic tube for a few weeks post-treatment. Penile and/or scrotal swelling is common in the first or second post-procedure weeks and usually resolves within 2 months of cryotherapy. Penile paraesthesia may occur and usually resolves within 2 to 4 months postprocedure. Long-term complications of cryotherapy include fistula formation, incontinence, erectile dysfunction, and urethral sloughing. The risk of permanent incontinence (i.e., need to wear a pad) is reported to range from < 1 to 8%. However, in individuals undergoing salvage cryotherapy after radiation failure, the incidence of urinary incontinence may be as high as 43%. Similarly, with total prostate gland cryotherapy, the ice ball extends beyond the capsule of the prostate and in most cases encompasses the neurovascular bundles and can cause erectile dysfunction. The incidence of erectile dysfunction after cryotherapy in the literature ranges from 49 to 93% at 1 year post-cryotherapy. The risk of fistula formation, a connection between the prostate and the rectum, occurs in 0 to 0.5% of individuals undergoing cryotherapy for prostate cancer and is highest in those men undergoing salvage cryotherapy after failed radiation therapy (EBRT). Urethral sloughing occurs less frequently with use of the urethral warming catheter. Urethral sloughing may cause dysuria and urinary retention. The incidence of urethral sloughing after cryotherapy with use of the urethral warming catheter ranges from 0 to 15%. Symptomatic patients may require transurethral resection of the necrotic tissue.

26. Are there different types of hormone therapy? Do I need to have my testicles removed?

Hormone therapy is a form of prostate cancer treatment designed to eliminate the male hormones (androgens) from the body. The most common androgen is **testosterone**. Androgens are primarily produced by the testicles, under control of various parts of the brain. A small number of androgens are produced by the adrenal glands, which are small glands located above the kidneys and produce many important chemicals. Prostate cancer cells may be hormone sensitive, hormone insensitive, or hormone resistant. Cancer cells that are hormone sensitive require androgens for growth. Thus, elimination of the androgens would prevent the growth of such cells and cause them to shrink. Normal prostate cells are also hormone sensitive and also shrink in response to hormone therapy. Prostate cancer cells that are hormone resistant continue to grow despite hormone therapy.

> **Testosterone**
>
> The male hormone or androgen that is produced primarily by the testes and is needed for sexual function and fertility.

> **Neoadjuvant therapy**
>
> The use of a treatment, such as chemotherapy, hormone therapy, and radiation therapy, before surgery.

Hormone therapy is not a curative therapy because it does not eliminate the prostate cancer cells; rather, it is palliative in that its goal is to slow down the progression, or growth, of the prostate cancer. Hormone therapy for patients with metastatic disease may work effectively for several years; however, over time, the hormone-resistant cells will emerge, and the cancer will grow.

Hormone therapy may be used as a primary, secondary, or **neoadjuvant therapy**. Hormone therapy is often used as a primary therapy in older men who are not candidates for surgery or radiation therapy and who are not interested in watchful waiting. It is also used in men who have metastatic disease at the time that their prostate cancer is detected. Men who experience a rise in their PSA after radical prostatectomy, radiation therapy, or

Hormone therapy is often used as a primary therapy in older men who are not candidates for surgery or radiation therapy and who are not interested in watchful waiting.

cryotherapy are given hormone therapy to slow down the growth of the recurrent prostate cancer. Lastly, hormone therapy may be given for a period of time before radical prostatectomy or radiation therapy to shrink the prostate gland and make the procedure easier to perform (neoadjuvant therapy). It is unclear whether this type of therapy affects the time to disease progression or survival. However, neoadjuvant therapy has a significant impact on the pathology, such that it is very difficult for the pathologist to grade the cancer cells after 3 months of hormone therapy.

In men with recurrent prostate cancer after EBRT or radical prostatectomy or in those who do not have organ-confined prostate cancer at the time of diagnosis, the time at which hormone therapy should be started is not clear. For this reason, one must weigh the potential benefits and side effects of hormone therapy. Hormone therapy may delay disease progression, but its effect on survival does not appear to be significant. In one study in men with prostate cancer, delaying hormone therapy for 1 year was associated with an 18% increase in the risk of death due to prostate cancer. Although this was a large study, it is still only one study, and more information is needed.

Many different forms of hormone therapy exist, both surgical therapy and medical therapy. The surgical approach is a bilateral **orchiectomy**, whereby the main source of androgen production, the testicles, are removed.

Orchiectomy

Removal of the testicle(s).

Bilateral orchiectomy is performed in men with prostate cancer to remove most of the testosterone production. Typically, this procedure can be performed as a minor surgical procedure under local anesthesia.

The advantages of bilateral orchiectomy are that it causes a quick drop in the testosterone level (the testosterone level drops to its lowest level by 3 to 12 hours after the procedure [average is 8.6 hours]), it is a one-time procedure, and it is more cost effective than the shots, which require several office visits per year and are more expensive. The disadvantages of orchiectomy are those of any surgical procedure and include bleeding, infection, permanence, and scrotal changes. In men who have undergone bilateral orchiectomy and are bothered by an empty scrotum, bilateral testicular prostheses may be placed that are the same size as the adult testes. Most men who undergo bilateral orchiectomy lose their libido and have erectile dysfunction after the testosterone level is lowered. Other long-term side effects of bilateral orchiectomy, related to testosterone depletion, include hot flashes, osteoporosis, fatigue, loss of muscle mass, anemia, and weight gain.

Medical therapy is designed to stop the production of androgens by the testicles. The three types of medical therapies are luteinizing hormone-releasing hormone (LHRH) analogues, antiandrogens, and gonadotropin-releasing hormone (GnRH) antagonists. These prevent the action of testosterone on the prostate cancer and on normal prostate cells (antiandrogen), or prevent the production of adrenal androgens.

Luteinizing Hormone-Releasing Hormone Analogues

The brain controls testosterone production by the testicles. Leuteinizing hormone-releasing hormone analogues are chemicals that stimulate the production of the luteinizing hormone, which tells the testicles to produce testosterone. Initially, when a man takes an LHRH analogue, there is an increased production of LH and of testosterone. This superstimulation tells the brain to stop producing LHRH and, subsequently, the testicles stop producing testosterone. It takes about 5 to 8 days for the LHRH analogues to drop the testosterone levels significantly. The increase in testosterone that sometimes occurs initially with LHRH analogues may affect patients with bone metastases, and there may be a worsening of their bone pain, which is called the **flare reaction**. Such men with metastatic disease will be given an antiandrogen before starting the LHRH analogue to prevent the flare phenomenon.

LHRH analogues are given as shots either monthly, every 3 months, every 4 months, every 6 months, or yearly. There are six forms of LHRH analogues: leuprolide acetate for intramuscular injection (Lupron Depot), triptorelin pamoate suspension for intramuscular injection (Trelstar Depot and Trelstar LA), leuprolide acetate for subcutaneous injection (Eligard), leuprolide acetate subcutaneous implant placement (Viadur), histrelin acetate for subcutaneous implant (Vantas), and goserelin acetate implant (Zoladex). They work in essentially the same way but differ in how they are given (**Table 8**). The advantage of this form of therapy is that it does not require removal of the testicles; however, it is expensive and requires more frequent visits to the doctor's office.

Intermittent hormone therapy is an alternative to standard hormone therapy. With intermittent hormone therapy you are treated for a period of time, usually until your PSA drops to a certain level, then the hormones are stopped until your PSA rises to a certain level. The idea of intermittent hormone therapy is that the prostate cancer cells that survive while you are on hormone therapy (hormone insensitive) become hormone sensitive again when they are exposed to androgens.

Flare reaction

A temporary increase in tumor growth and symptoms that is caused by the initial use of LHRH agonists. It is prevented by the use of an antiandrogen one week before LHRH agonist therapy begins.

Prostate Cancer

Table 8   Commonly Used Antiandrogens, LHRH Analogues and Antagonists

Agent	Dose	Route of Administration	Action	Side Effects
Lupron Depot (leuprolide acetate for depot injection)	7.5 mg/mo 22.5 mg/3 mos 30 mg/4 mos	IM	LHRH analogue	Impotence, decreased libido, osteoporosis, anemia, hot flashes, weight gain, fatigue, flare phenomenon
Eligard (leuprolide acetate for injectable suspension)	7.5 mg/mo 22.5 mg/3 mos 30 mg/4 mos 45 mg/6 mos	SQ	LHRH analogue	Same as Lupron
Trelstar Depot/LA (triptorelin pamoate injectable suspension)	3.75 mg/mo 11.25 mg/3 mos	IM	LHRH analogue	Same as Lupron
Vantas (histrelin acetate implant)	50 mg/yr	SQ	LHRH analogue	Same as Lupron
Viadur (leuprolide acetate)	65 mg/yr	SQ implant—requires incision for placement	LHRH analogue	Same as Lupron
Zoladex (goserelin)	3.6 mg/mo 10.8 mg/3 mos	SQ	LHRH analogue	Same as Lupron

(Continued)

Table 8 Commonly Used Antiandrogens, LHRH Analogues and Antagonists (*Continued*)

Agent	Dose	Route of Administration	Action	Side Effects
Firmagon (degarelix)	240 mg given as two injections of 120 mg each as initial dose followed 28 days later by maintenance dose of 80 mg Q28 days	SQ	LHRH antagonist	Injection site reactions, hot flash, impotence, weight gain, fatigue, increase in transaminases, HTN, chills
Eulexin (flutamide)	750 mg/day	PO	Antiandrogen	Breast tenderness and enlargement, hot flashes, diarrhea, anemia, abnormal liver function
Nilandron (nilutamide)	300 mg/day 3 3 1 mo	PO	Antiandrogen	Same as with Eulexin. Also, reversible lung disease, alcohol intolerance, decreased night vision
Casodex (bicalutamide) comb rx	50 mg/day	PO	Antiandrogen	Same as with Eulexin

Abbreviations: mos, months; PO, orally; SQ, subcutaneously; comb rx, combination treatment; IM, intramuscularly.

Possible advantages of intermittent androgen suppression include preservation of androgen sensitivity of the tumor, possible prolonged survival, improved quality of life because of recovery of libido and potency and improved sense of well-being, decrease in treatment costs, increased sensitivity of the prostate cancer to chemotherapy, and the fact that it can be used to treat all stages of prostate cancer. Intermittent hormone therapy appears to affect bone mineral density loss at 6 years.

The long-term effects of intermittent hormone therapy are not well known. The duration of the hormone therapy, the best time to restart hormone therapy, how to tell whether the disease is progressing, and who is the ideal patient for intermittent hormone therapy are not well defined. One potential way to give intermittent androgen suppression therapy (androgen blockade) is shown in **Table 9**.

LHRH analogues often are used alone as primary, secondary, or neoadjuvant therapy. Over time, the PSA level may increase. When the PSA increases, your doctor may check your serum testosterone level to make sure that the LHRH analogue is dropping the testosterone level to almost undetectable levels. In some cases with use of the LHRH analogue on an every-3-to 4-month basis, the testosterone suppression may not be adequate, and switching to a more frequent dosing interval, such as an every 28-day formulation, may be more effective. When a man is receiving hormone therapy, the testosterone level should be < 20 ng/dL. When the PSA increases despite LHRH analogues, the LHRH analogues are continued, and another medication, an antiandrogen, is added. This combined therapy is called

Table 9   Intermittent Androgen Blockage

PSA nadir < 4 ng/mL
Continue on therapy for an average of 9 months
↓
Discontinue medications
Watch until PSA increases to mean of 10–20 ng/mL
↓
Resume total androgen blockade
Continue cycling until regulation of PSA becomes independent of total androgen blockade

Ellsworth, P. *100 Questions and Answers About Prostate Cancer*, 2e. Jones and Bartlett Publishers, LLC, 2009.

total androgen blockade and is often effective in treating the prostate cancer for 3 to 6 months.

Antiandrogens

Antiandrogens are receptor blockers; they prevent the attachment of the androgens, both those produced by the testicles and those produced by the adrenal glands, to the prostate cancer cells, thus preventing them from acting on these cells. Because these chemicals do not actually affect testosterone production, the testosterone level remains normal or may be slightly elevated if they are used alone. Thus, these medications do not affect libido or erectile function when used alone. However, antiandrogens are more commonly used in combination with LHRH analogues. One antiandrogen, bicalutamide (Casodex) is approved for use as a monotherapy in Europe but has not been approved by the FDA.

Antiandrogen

Drugs that counteract the action of testosterone.

There are three commonly used antiandrogens: bicalutamide (Casodex), flutamide (Eulexin), and nilutamide
(Nilandron) (Table 8). As with all medications, these
have side effects, which are listed in Table 8. When
antiandrogens are used in combination with LHRH
analogues, this is called **total androgen blockade**. Total
androgen blockade is used for individuals whose PSA
increases significantly while they are taking LHRH
analogues.

Newer Therapies

Aberelix is a **GnRH antagonist**. Unlike the LHRH
agonists, the GnRH antagonist does not initially cause
an increase in testosterone level. Instead, it works to
decrease testosterone more quickly. Aberelix can cause
serious and life-threatening allergic reactions and therefore it is no longer available for use in the treatment of
prostate cancer. Patients who have been previously
prescribed by doctors enrolled in a special program, the
Plenaxis PLUS Program, can continue to receive Aberelix
as long as they continue to do well with the medication.

Degarelix is an LHRH antagonist which has been
demonstrated in clinical trials to rapidly decrease serum
testosterone (within 3 days) and is not associated with
the initial surge of testosterone and risk of flare that is
seen with LHRH agonists. It has been recently approved
by the FDA. The starting dose is 240 mg given as two
subcutaneous injections of 120 mg, then maintenance
doses of 80 mg as one subcutaneous injection every 28
days. Phase III studies have demonstrated that degarelix
is at least as effective as leuprolide (Lupron Depot®) in
sustaining castrate levels or lower of testosterone and
had a statistically significant faster decrease in testosterone levels.

Degarelix is an LHRH antagonist which has been demonstrated in clinical trials to rapidly decrease serum testosterone (within 3 days) and is not associated with the initial surge of testosterone and risk of flare that is seen with GnRH agonist.

Prostate Cancer

27. What are some of the side effects of hormonal therapy and how are they treated?

LHRH analogues and antagonists have side effects that may affect your quality of life over the short and long term (Table 9). Some of the side effects related to these medications, such as hot flashes, erectile dysfunction, anemia, and osteoporosis, can be treated. Erectile dysfunction occurs in about 80% of men taking LHRH analogues and antagonists and is associated with decreased libido (sexual desire). The widely prescribed drug sildenafil (Viagra) as well as the other oral therapies for erectile dysfunction, vardenafil (Levitra) and tadalafil (Cialis) are effective in most of these men if they had normal erectile function before starting hormone therapy. Unfortunately, there is no medication to restore libido.

A recent Gallup survey of American men revealed that most men believe that osteoporosis is "a woman's disease." **Osteoporosis** is loss of bone density, and it leads to weakened bones that break more easily. Yet this disease can affect men, particularly men taking hormone therapy for prostate cancer. It is anticipated that there will be approximately 2,000 osteoporosis-induced fractures in men with advanced prostate cancer.

How can you tell if you have osteoporosis? The best way to check the bone mineral density is the dual-energy x-ray absorptiometry (DEXA) scan, the same study used to evaluate for osteoporosis in women. It is noninvasive, precise, and a quick test involving minimal radiation exposure. The test measures the bone mineral density, which is compared with values obtained from normal, young, adult control subjects.

Several factors contribute to loss of bone mineral density, but decreased sex hormone production has the most

Osteoporosis

The reduction in the amount of bone mass, leading to fractures after minimal trauma.

significant impact on bone mineral density. Low testosterone levels affect bone mineral density in men almost the same as low estrogen levels in women. The use of androgen deprivation therapy, whether it is via orchiectomy or LHRH analogue or LHRH antagonist with or without antiandrogen, causes decreased bone mineral density. There is an average loss of 4% per year for the first 2 years on hormone therapy and 2% per year after year 4, which is similar to the loss in women after removal of the ovaries or natural menopause. This loss of bone mineral density in men taking hormone therapy occurs for at least ten years and probably accounts for the increased incidence of fractures: 5 to 13.5% of men taking hormone therapy have fractures compared to 1% in men with prostate cancer who are not receiving hormone therapy.

Lifestyle modifications that may help decrease the risks of bone complications in men on hormonal therapy include smoking cessation, decreased alcohol intake, performing weight bearing and arm exercises, and taking supplements of 1200 mg of calcium and 400 to 800 international units of vitamin D daily. Calcium rich diets include dairy products, salmon, spinach, and tofu.

When should men on hormone therapy be evaluated for osteoporosis? There are no good guidelines to help determine how frequently DEXA scans should be obtained in men with prostate cancer who are taking hormone therapy. It may be helpful to obtain a baseline DEXA scan before starting hormone therapy and then obtain periodic DEXA scans thereafter. There are things that can be done to prevent or treat osteoporosis. Several studies have shown that an increase in bone mineral density loss occurs in men who have had an orchiectomy compared to men who are receiving LHRH analogues. The reason for this is not clear, but this result suggests that other

It may be helpful to obtain a baseline DEXA scan before starting hormone therapy and then obtain periodic DEXA scans thereafter.

chemicals are produced by the testes that may be important in maintaining bone density. Further studies may help identify these chemicals. Certain factors can put one at increased risk for osteoporosis, including sedentary lifestyle, decreased sun exposure, glucocorticoid therapy, excess caffeine intake, decreased dietary calcium and vitamin D intake or exposure, increased salt intake, aluminum-containing antacid consumption, alcohol abuse, and smoking.

Changes in lifestyle can help prevent osteoporosis. Various medications have been used in women with osteoporosis, but no treatments have been approved by the United States Food and Drug Administration (FDA) for men taking hormone therapy.

A group of medications commonly used in women with osteoporosis are the biphosphonates, which prevent bone breakdown. Three different biphosphonates, aledronate (Fosamax), neridronate (Nerexia), and zoledronate (Zometa) have been used to prevent osteoporosis in androgen-deficient men with prostate cancer. Zoledronate has been shown to increase bone density in men on hormonal therapy. Intermittent administration of either intravenous pamidronate or zoledronic acid prevents treatment-related bone loss in men with prostate cancer. In a clinical study, zoledronic acid (4 mg intravenous every 3 months) prevented bone loss and actually increased bone marrow density, during androgen-deprivation therapy for prostate cancer. Side effects of intravenous biphosphonates include an influenza-like illness (14–15%), hot flashes (23–58%), fatigue (10–38%), arthralgias (13–22%) and fever (10–11.5%). Osteonecrosis of the jaw (ONJ) has been reported in cancer patients receiving complex treatment regimens, including radiation therapy, chemotherapy, and/or corticosteroids, along with an intravenous biphosphonate. ONJ has been reported more frequently in patients with cancer types other than prostate cancer. Cancer patients undergoing invasive dental procedures (i.e. tooth extraction) are at greater risk of developing ONJ.

Another way of decreasing the risk of osteoporosis is the use of intermittent hormone therapy. With this form of therapy, you are on and off the hormones for set periods of time. The idea of intermittent hormone therapy is that the prostate cancer cells that survive while you are on hormone therapy (hormone insensitive) become hormone sensitive again when they are exposed to androgens. Possible advantages of intermittent androgen suppression include preservation of androgen sensitivity of the tumor, possible prolonged survival, improved quality of life because of recovery of libido and potency and improved sense of well-being, decrease in treatment costs, increased sensitivity of the prostate cancer to chemotherapy, and the fact that it can be used to treat all stages of prostate cancer. Intermittent hormone therapy appears to affect bone mineral density loss at six years.

Hot Flushes/Flashes

Hot flashes occur in men receiving hormone therapy for the treatment of high-stage prostate cancer and in patients receiving neoadjuvant hormone therapy (hormone therapy administered before definitive treatment, e.g., radical prostatectomy or interstitial seeds to shrink the prostate cancer).

Approximately three-quarters (75%) of the men being treated with hormone therapy for prostate cancer report bothersome hot flashes that begin 1 to 12 months after starting hormone therapy and often persist for years. The hot flashes may vary in intensity and can last from a few seconds to an hour.

The cause of hot flashes and sweating (vasomotor symptoms) associated with hormone therapy (shots or orchiectomy) is not well known. The symptoms are similar to those that women experience while going through menopause, yet they are not typically experienced by men, whose testosterone level slowly declines with aging. The symptoms appear to be related to the sudden large decrease in the testosterone level and the effects that testosterone has on blood vessels. There are no identifiable factors that put one individual at higher risk for hot flashes than another.

There are many ways to treat hot flashes associated with hormone therapy, and different men respond to different treatments (**Table 10**). Some options include clonidine (a blood pressure medication), the hormone megestrol acetate (Megace), medroxyprogesterone acetate (Provera), estrogen patches, low-dose estrogen (DES), and medroxyprogesterone acetate (Depo-Provera). Oral estrogen has been effective in getting rid of the hot flashes; however, estrogen use carries the risk of heart problems, strokes, and blood clots. Low-dose megestrol acetate (Megace) has been used effectively to treat hot flashes and works in about 85% of people. However, it has been associated in rare cases with an increase in PSA that decreased with stopping the Megace and must be used cautiously. Another chemical, cyproterone acetate, has been used to treat hot flashes, but it is associated with cardiac side effects, is expensive, and is not approved for this use by the FDA. The hormone Provera, given orally or intramuscularly, has been effective in treating hot flashes, but it also may have

Table 10   Drugs Commonly Used in Treating Hot Flashes

Drug	Dosage	Possible Side Effects
Megestrol acetate (Megace)	20 mg BID	Chills, appetite stimulation, weight gain
Clonidine (Catapres)	0.1-mg patch each week	Hypotension, skin reaction
Medroxyprogesterone Acetate (Provera or Depo-Provera)	400 mg IM or 25 mg PO BID	Cardiovascular side effects
Venlafaxine	12.5 mg PO BID	Depression, nausea, loss of appetite
Cyproterone acetate	50 mg PO TID	Rarely, tumor may grow; cardiovascular side effects
Diethylstilbestrol (DES)	1 mg PO QD	Cardiovascular side effects, difficult to obtain, blood clots

Abbreviations: BID, twice a day; TID, three times a day; IM, intramuscularly; PO, orally; QD, every day.

Ellsworth, P. *100 Questions and Answers About Prostate Cancer*, 2e. Jones and Bartlett Publishers, LLC, 2009.

some cardiovascular side effects. Clonidine patches have been helpful in decreasing the incidence and severity of hot flashes with natural or surgically-induced (hysterectomy and removal of the ovaries) menopause, but they do not appear to be as effective in men. Eating a serving of soy daily in addition to 800 IU of vitamin E in one study was shown to decrease the number and the severity of hot flashes to 50% (see Question 9). You should not take this amount of vitamin E without consulting your doctor first. Lastly, antidepressants such as gabapentin and venlafaxine have been shown to be useful in treating hot flashes. Limiting caffeine intake and avoiding strenuous exercise and very warm temperatures are also helpful in controlling hot flashes.

Breast Swelling and Tenderness (Gynecomastia)

Antiandrogens may cause swelling and tenderness in the breast area (gynecomastia). This can affect one or both breasts and can range from mild sensitivity to ongoing pain. About one-half of men taking antiandrogens will develop breast swelling and between 25% and 75% will note some breast tenderness. Gynecomastia is not as common in men who have had an orchiectomy or in those who are on combination therapy (an LHRH agonist or antagonist and an anti-androgen). A single dose of radiation to the breasts can decrease the risk of developing gynecomastia but is only effective if the radiation is given the first month of the hormone therapy. If gynecomastia has already developed then radiation treatment is not helpful. Tamoxifen, a medication that is used to treat breast cancer, can help in treating gynecomastia in men taking antiandrogens. It can't be used in those men who are taking estrogens (DES) to treat prostate cancer as the tamoxifen stops the estrogens from working properly. Tamoxifen may help treat gynecomastia that has already developed in men after starting antiandrogens. Another option for the treatment of gynecomastia is surgical removal of the breast tissue. However, this has the risk of damage to the nipple and loss of feeling.

Hormone therapy can also cause weight gain and muscle loss. Exercise and diet regimens can help with these problems. Hormone therapy can also cause tiredness and lethargy, memory problems, and moodiness. The lethargy and tiredness may improve over time, but regular exercise can give men more energy and help them cope.

Anemia (lowering of the red blood cell count) may occur in men who are on hormone therapy. For men with advanced prostate cancer, use of an LHRH agonist/antagonist without the antiandrogen may be beneficial in limiting the anemia that is caused by complete androgen blockade (antiandrogen plus LHRH agonist or antagonist). Erythropoietin, iron preparations, and vitamin supplementation may be helpful in improving the anemia.

28. What happens when hormone therapy fails?

If the PSA level increases while you are receiving total androgen blockade (LHRH agonist or antagonist plus androgen receptor blocker), first your doctor will stop the antiandrogen, which is called antiandrogen withdrawal (**Figure 19**). This causes the PSA to decrease in about 20% of patients, and the effect may last for several months to years. The LHRH analogue/antagonist therapy is continued. It is not clear why this antiandrogen withdrawal works. When the PSA rises after antiandrogen withdrawal, you may consider other forms of hormone therapy, such as ketoconazole, aminoglutethimide, estrogens, progestins, another antiandrogen, and chemotherapy.

Aminoglutethimide has produced a decrease in PSA in 48 to 80% of patients when it is given with a steroid (hydrocortisone) at the time of antiandrogen withdrawal. Side effects of aminoglutethimide include lowering of the blood pressure when you stand up (orthostatic hypotension), fatigue, gait disturbance (ataxia), and skin rash.

Ketoconazole is a medication that decreases androgen production from both the testicles and the adrenal glands and also works directly on the prostate cancer cells. In patients who have not responded to first-line hormone therapy (LHRH analogue or antagonist plus antiandrogen), Ketoconazole plus hydrocortisone decreases the PSA in about 15% of patients. In those who have not

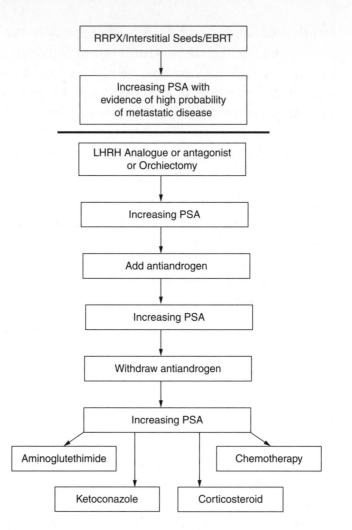

Figure 19 Treatment of increasing PSA after primary therapy (RRPX/ interstitial seeds/EBRT).

Ketoconazole works quickly; its effects on testosterone level start 30 minutes after it is taken, and the testosterone level is decreased by 90% within 48 hours after therapy is started.

responded to antiandrogen withdrawal, ketoconazole plus hydrocortisone decreases PSA in about 75% of men.

Ketoconazole works quickly; its effects on testosterone level start 30 minutes after it is taken, and the testosterone level is decreased by 90% within 48 hours after therapy is started. The usual dose is 200 mg three times a day for the first week and then 400 mg orally three times a day thereafter. Some men respond to a lower dose of 200 mg three times a day as long-term therapy. The recommended dose of hydrocortisone is 20 mg at breakfast and 20 mg at dinner. If you develop ankle swelling or worsening of diabetes, then the dose is decreased to 20 mg in the morning and 10 mg in the evening, or simply 10 mg twice a day.

Side effects of ketoconazole include nausea and vomiting in about 15% of patients. Ideally, it should be taken between meals and not with antacids, Carafate, histamine^2 blockers (ranitidine [Zantac], cimetidine [Tagamet], famotidine [Pepcid], nizatidine [Axid]), or protein pump inhibitors (omeprazole [Prilosec], lansoprazole [Prevacid], Nexus). It can also increase liver function blood abnormalities but rarely causes actual liver problems. Blood should be drawn to check the liver function regularly while you are taking ketoconazole. Ketoconazole has the potential to interact with other medications that are metabolized by the liver, so check with your doctor if you are taking multiple medications to make sure that you are not taking anything that will have an interaction.

Corticosteroids (e.g., prednisone) can also decrease the production of androgens by the adrenal gland. They also have beneficial effects on appetite and energy level. Decreases in PSA have occurred in 20 to 29% of patients with **hormone-refractory** prostate cancer who are taking corticosteroids. Other corticosteroids, such as dexamethasone and megestrol acetate, may also improve symptoms.

Hormone refractory

Prostate cancer that is resistant to hormone therapy.

Chemotherapy has an increasing role in the management of men with hormone refractory/resistant prostate cancer. **Docetaxel**, a chemotherapeutic drug approved for hormone refractory prostate cancer, has been shown to increase survival with manageable side effects in men with hormone refractory prostate cancer, when compared

Docetaxel

A type of chemotherapy, a taxane, that has been shown to be effective in hormone refractory prostate cancer.

to other forms of chemotherapy. The positive response noted with docetaxel has promoted researchers to evaluate additional chemotherapeutic drugs in ongoing clinical trials. Such trials allow some patients to participate in evaluating the effectiveness and safety of newer forms of chemotherapy. They may or may not prove to be beneficial for the participant, but the information gained from them allows oncologists to learn more about prostate cancer and effective treatment options. If you are interested in clinical trials, talk to your doctor about this or contact your local cancer center.

Provenge (produced by Dendreon) is an experimental vaccine therapy for advanced prostate cancer. Provenge is developed from one's own blood. A sample of blood is withdrawn and processed to extract certain immune cells called antigen presenting cells (APCs). Protein and prostatic acid phosphatase (PHP), found in most cancers, are then mixed. The prostate acid phosphatase is fused with an immune stimulating substance called GM-CSF. The mixture is then infused back into the patient over an hour's duration. This is repeated three times over the course of a month. Recent study results have demonstrated that those patients with advanced prostate cancer who received Provenge immunotherapy lived 4 months longer than patients with advanced prostate cancer receiving placebo in the trial.

29. What happens if my PSA rises after radical prostatectomy? After external beam radiation therapy (EBRT)? After interstitial seed therapy?

When the PSA rises after definitive therapy, such as EBRT, interstitial seed therapy, and radical prostatectomy, it is called PSA progression. In the absence of any identifiable cancer, it is called biochemical progression, because the only indicator of progression of the cancer is the PSA level. When the PSA is increasing after definitive therapy, your physician may want to restage you to determine where the cancer is. It is helpful in the decision-making process to determine whether the prostate cancer is confined to the prostate (in men who have had interstitial seed therapy or EBRT), the area where the prostate was (in postradical-prostatectomy patients), or the pelvis, or whether it has spread outside of the prostatic area. For example, if it has spread to the bones or lymph nodes higher up in your abdomen. Methods used in this staging process may be a bone scan (see Question 12), a ProstaScint scan, and/or a CT scan of the abdomen and pelvis. In certain cases, the doctor may recommend a biopsy of the prostate, of the bladder neck area, or of other areas that may be likely to have cancer.

After a radical prostatectomy your PSA should decrease to an undetectable level by approximately 4 weeks postoperative. However, a detectable PSA level after this time does not mean that there is necessarily clinically significant recurrent prostate cancer. Some patients with a detectable PSA after radical prostatectomy do not have progression of their cancer because the PSA level is the result of the presence of benign prostate tissue at the margins of the resection (a very small amount of benign prostate tissue being left behind) or from a dormant residual focus of prostate cancer at a local or distant site. The definition of biochemical recurrence (evidence of recurrent prostate cancer based on PSA testing only) varies from a PSA of 0.2 ng/ml to 0.4 ng/ml post radical prostatectomy. In a large number of patients a biochemical recurrence of 0.2 is associated with a slowly progressive course.

Your doctor will look at a variety of factors to determine if the rising PSA is caused by benign tissue left behind at the time of surgery, locally recurrent prostate cancer that is amenable to radiation therapy, or metastatic prostate cancer that will require hormone therapy. Several investigators have looked at various criteria that may help distinguish local recurrence from distant metastases for patients with a rising PSA after radical prostatectomy. A Gleason score 8–10, seminal vesicle invasion, positive lymph nodes and a rapid PSA velocity (rate of change of the PSA) and a short disease-free interval after radical prostatectomy have been associated with a greater chance of metastatic disease.

Overall, about 35% of men who have had a radical prostatectomy will experience a detectable serum PSA within 10 years after surgery. The risk of developing metastatic disease after biochemical recurrence correlates with pathologic Gleason scores. Men with tumors of Gleason score < 8 have a 73% chance of remaining free of progression at 5 years after biochemical recurrence, compared with a < 10% probability in men with high grade tumors (Gleason 8–10). The length of time after surgery prior to biochemical recurrence was important in determining the risk of eventual distant failure for men with lower (5–7) and men with higher (8–10) Gleason scores. Using a cutoff of 10 months, the prostate specific antigen doubling time (PSADT) provides further substratification for men with Gleason scores of < 8. Men with a rapid rise in PSA (shorter PSA doubling time) have a greater risk of metastatic disease.

Several options are available, including watchful waiting, salvage EBRT, and hormone therapy.

Salvage Radiation Therapy

In males with a rising PSA after radical prostatectomy in whom the disease is felt to be locally recurrent, rather than metastatic, salvage radiation therapy is an option. The ASTRO (American Society for Therapeutic Radiology and Oncology) consensus panel concluded that the appropriate PSA seemed to be 1.5ng/ml for the institution of salvage radiation therapy. Others have demonstrated improved outcomes using a PSA threshold of 0.6. Gleason score 8–10, pre-radiotherapy PSA level > 2.0, negative surgical margin, PSA doubling time of 10 months or less, and seminal vesicle invasion are significant predictors of disease progression despite salvage radiation therapy. Conversely, a positive surgical margin suggests a greater likelihood that the recurrence is due to residual pelvic disease, therefore a patient with a history of a positive margin who develops an increasing PSA is most likely to benefit from salvage radiation therapy.

If your disease is metastatic, you are not a candidate or you are not interested in salvage radiation therapy, your doctor will discuss with you the options of watchful-waiting and hormone therapy.

Watchful Waiting

In one study, watchful waiting was used in men with a rising PSA after radical prostatectomy, and they were monitored until they had evidence of metastases. About 8 years after the radical prostatectomy, these men developed metastases, and an additional 5 years later, they died from their prostate cancer. In general, when watchful waiting is used for PSA progression after radical prostatectomy, the PSA is checked on an every 3 to 6 month basis to determine how quickly the PSA is rising (PSA velocity). If the doubling time, the time that it takes for

In general, when watchful waiting is used for PSA progression after radical prostatectomy, the PSA is checked on an every 3 to 6 month basis to determine how quickly the PSA is rising (PSA velocity).

the PSA level to double, is long (a year or longer), then the tumor is slow growing. If the doubling time is short (every 3 months), then the tumor is fast growing, and the patient would probably benefit from early treatment as opposed to continuing with watchful waiting.

Hormone Therapy

Hormone therapy tends to be used more commonly for men with recurrent cancer in whom the recurrence is believed to be outside of the pelvic area. Although hormone therapy may delay the progression of the prostate cancer, its impact on survival in this situation is not well known. Men with high-grade tumors (Gleason sum > 7) or with cancer in the seminal vesicles or lymph nodes at the time of radical prostatectomy and in whom the PSA rises within 2 years after prostatectomy most likely have distant disease and are candidates for hormone therapy or watchful waiting.

What if the PSA rises after EBRT?

Historically, three consecutive PSA rises after achieving a PSA nadir was felt to be indicative of biochemical recurrence after EBRT. However, in 2005, a consensus panel meeting was held, which concluded that a PSA value of 2 ng/mL greater than the absolute nadir represents the best revised definition of failure following external-beam radiation monotherapy. In individuals with biochemical failure after EBRT, the options of treatment include salvage prostatectomy, salvage cryotherapy, hormone therapy, and watchful waiting. The decision regarding the most appropriate therapy is based on the likelihood of the cancer being confined to the prostate.

Salvage Prostatectomy after EBRT

The ideal patient for a salvage radical prostatectomy after EBRT is one who is believed to have had prostate-confined disease initially at the time of EBRT and who is still believed to have organ-confined disease. Individuals in this group include those who have a Gleason score ≤ 6, a low pretreatment PSA level (< 10 ng/mL), and low clinical stage tumor (T1c or T2a). At the time of the salvage prostatectomy, they should still have a favorable Gleason score, a low clinical stage, and, ideally, a PSA that is < 4 ng/mL. Salvage prostatectomy is a challenging procedure, and if you are considering this option, you should seek out an urologist who has experience with it because there is an increased risk of urinary incontinence, erectile dysfunction, and rectal injury with this procedure. Rarely, because of extensive scarring, it is necessary to remove the bladder in addition to the prostate, and a urinary diversion would be necessary. A urinary diversion is a procedure that allows urine to be diverted to a segment of bowel that can be made into a storage unit similar to a bladder or allows urine to pass out of an opening in the belly wall into a bag, similar to a colostomy.

Salvage Cryotherapy

One of the main uses of cryotherapy is in patients with a rising PSA after EBRT. In patients who have not responded locally to EBRT, approximately 40% who then undergo salvage cryotherapy will have an undetectable PSA level after cryotherapy, and 78% will have negative prostate biopsy results. It appears that a drop in the PSA to ≤ 0.5 ng/mL after cryotherapy is associated with a good prognosis. In men with postcryotherapy PSA levels > 0.5 ng/mL, there is a higher likelihood that the PSA will increase or that the prostate biopsy result will be positive.

Hormone Therapy and Watchful Waiting

Use of these two options in patients with a rising PSA after EBRT is similar to their use in those with a rising PSA after radical prostatectomy.

Treatment of Rising PSA after Interstitial Seed Therapy

Treatment options for a rising PSA after interstitial seed therapy include salvage prostatectomy, EBRT, watchful waiting, and hormone therapy. It is important to remember that after interstitial seed therapy, there may be a benign rise in the PSA level, and this should not be misconstrued as being indicative of recurrent prostate cancer. In both interstitial seed and radiation therapy, for a rising PSA to be indicative of recurrent/persistent prostate cancer, it must rise sequentially on three occasions at least two weeks apart. The treatment options are dependent on the likelihood of the disease being confined to the prostate. Salvage prostatectomy for interstitial seed failure carries the same risks as with EBRT failures. The ability to use EBRT depends on the amount of radiation that was delivered at the time of the interstitial seeds and the likelihood of the disease being confined to the prostate.

30. What happens if I develop bone pain?

When prostate cancer metastasizes, it tends to travel to the pelvic lymph nodes first and then to the bones. Bone metastases may be silent, meaning that they do not cause any pain, or they may be symptomatic, causing pain or leading to a fracture. Bone metastases are typically identified on a bone scan and can also be seen on a plain X-ray.

There are many ways to treat bone pain. Your doctor will likely try the simplest treatments and those associated with the least side effects first, and then progress as needed. Nonsteroidal anti-inflammatories, such as ibuprofen, are typically used as a first-line treatment. If the pain is not controlled with these, then narcotics, such as Tylenol with codeine, are added. For patients with a localized bone metastasis that is causing persistent discomfort, localized radiation therapy may be used

(XRT is not useful for men with multiple bone metastases). XRT provides pain relief in 80 to 90% of patients, and the relief may last for up to 1 year in slightly more than half of these men. Usually, the total radiation dose is given over 5 to 15 quick treatment sessions.

When multiple painful bone metastases are present, hemibody radiation may be used. Because this therapy affects a larger area of the body, there are more side effects, including lowering of the blood pressure (hypotension), nausea, vomiting, diarrhea, lung irritation, hair loss, and lowering of the blood count. Hemibody radiation is also given over several treatment sessions. It can lead to pain control that lasts up to one year in as many as 70% of individuals.

Another form of therapy for multiple painful bone metastasis is radioisotope therapy. With this form of therapy, a radioisotope, a chemical with a radioactive component, is injected into a vein. The chemicals used preferentially go to bone that is affected by cancer. These chemicals are picked up by the bone and radiate the area. Two such agents are strontium 89 and samarium 153.

Another form of therapy for multiple painful bone metastasis is radioisotope therapy.

Strontium 89 is a chemical similar to calcium and tends to concentrate in areas of the body where calcium is absorbed, such as bone, and it preferentially goes to areas of bone metastases. Only a small amount of the injected dose remains in the bones after 1 week and most is eliminated in the urine. For this reason, it is important to carefully dispose of urine for the first week after injection. The strontium 89 that is picked up by the bones will exert its radiation effect for as many as 50 days, whereas in normal bone it is effective for only about 14 days. During this time, you are not considered a radiation hazard to friends or family.

Strontium 89 (Metastron) improves bone pain in 80 to 86% of individuals, and relief starts about 2 weeks after treatment. However, pain relief may be preceded by an initial increase in pain. Strontium 89 has also been used in combination with EBRT. In patients receiving both therapies, there is no apparent increase in survival. Those who receive the combination therapy have a decreased need for pain medications and an increase in physical activity, fewer sites of new bone pain requiring palliative EBRT, and larger decreases in PSA. Studies are being performed to evaluate the effect of combining strontium 89 with various forms of chemotherapy, such as doxorubicin (Adriamycin).

Because strontium 89 does affect normal bone, albeit to a lesser degree than that affected by prostate cancer, blood counts must be monitored because the bone is responsible for producing the blood cells. Typically, the blood counts are checked twice a week, but more frequently if needed. If the platelet and white blood cell counts are stable, you may be retreated with strontium 89, if needed.

Another radioisotope is samarium 153 (Quadramet). It is a newer agent that is also administered intravenously. It has been shown to be effective in decreasing bone pain and produces a mild decrease in the blood count.

Biphosphonates are chemicals that interfere with bone breakdown and are typically used for treatment of osteoporosis. Most prostate cancer bone metastases are not lytic metastases (i.e., they do not cause bone breakdown), but some bone breakdown does appear to occur; biphosphonates lead to improvement in bone symptoms in men with prostate cancer. Their use in bone pain remains investigational.

PART TWO

Benign Prostatic Hyperplasia (BPH)

What causes BPH?

When does BPH need to be treated and what are the treatment options?

What is laser treatment and what types are available?

More . . .

31. What causes BPH?

The short answer is that no one knows for sure. The growth of the prostate gland is a complex process that starts at puberty and continues throughout adult life. As a man ages, his prostate grows, although the rate of growth and size of the prostate varies from individual to individual. It is certain that prostate growth, whether it is benign or malignant, requires testosterone and a derivative of testosterone, dihydrotestosterone. Centuries ago, it was observed that the castrati, the Italian opera singers who were castrated at puberty to preserve their tenor voices, never developed enlargement of their prostates.

32. How common is BPH?

BPH is the most common disease of mankind. It has been said that if a man lives long enough, he will develop BPH; however, autopsy studies have shown that some men, even in their 30s, have anatomic evidence for significant prostate enlargement. The degree of prostatic enlargement is variable; however, the following numbers are useful guidelines. At the age of 30 years, an average prostate size is 20 grams; by age 70 years, the average prostate size is 35 grams.

As an estimate, if you take a man's chronologic age in years, roughly that percentage of men at that age will have signs of BPH. It is important to note that there is not a linear correlation between prostate size and prostate symptoms. Some men with relatively small glands will have significant symptoms, whereas some men with large glands will have minimal symptoms.

33. What are the symptoms of BPH?

An enlarged prostate can cause a variety of symptoms. Some are referred to as obstructive/voiding symptoms and include weak stream, hesitancy of voiding, intermittent stream, a sensation of incomplete bladder emptying, and terminal dribbling. Storage/irritative symptoms include frequent urination, nocturia (getting up at night to urinate), and urgency, the sudden compelling need to urinate that is difficult to defer. These storage symptoms are overactive bladder symptoms.

Other conditions that may be a sign of prostatic enlargement are urinary retention or the inability to void, urinary tract infection, urinary incontinence, and hematuria or blood in the urine.

It is important to acknowledge that bladder dysfunction can either mimic or contribute to some of these symptoms, and the physician must consider these when a diagnosis of prostatic enlargement is made.

34. How is BPH diagnosed?

Both a physical exam and history are used to diagnose BPH. When necessary, the urologist may use other diagnostic tests to obtain additional information to help make the diagnosis.

If a patient gives a history that includes one or more of the symptoms mentioned in Question 33, the physician will be alerted to consider BPH as part of his differential diagnosis. Also, when the physician performs a digital rectal exam (palpates or feels the prostate with a finger in the rectum), he or she can feel whether the prostate is enlarged. Your doctor may ask you to complete a simple screening tool called the AUA symptom score, although it is not specific for BPH, it allows the doctor to determine the severity of your symptoms and may provide a way of assessing whether or not your symptoms have improved with treatment. This symptom score has been adopted worldwide with the addition of a question pertaining to quality of life and is referred to as the International Prostate Symptom Score (IPSS) (**Figure 20**).

Finally, if the physician needs additional information before making a diagnosis of BPH, he or she can do additional tests.

What tests may be involved with the diagnosis of BPH?

Not everyone with lower urinary tract symptoms (LUTs) suggestive of BPH will require special tests to make a diagnosis. However, in certain individuals further testing may be helpful in guiding the management.

Uroflow: A uroflow measurement is a totally noninvasive test. The patient, with a full bladder, voids into a special urinal that has a flowmeter, which measures both the urine flow in milliliters per second as well as the total volume voided. This is plotted onto a piece of paper, and there are nomograms available that allow the doctor to compare the patient's urine flow rate with accepted standards. The uroflow is typically done in the physician's office at the time of the patient's visit. A low urine flow rate is suggestive, but not definitive, for bladder outlet obstruction, which may be caused by BPH or a urethral stricture. However, in the individual whose bladder does not contract adequately, the urine flow rate may also be low. The urine flow rate can also look better than it really is if you push with your abdominal muscles while voiding. Thus, although helpful, it is not entirely accurate.

Bladder ultrasound/scanner PVR: A bladder ultrasound is performed by placing an ultrasound probe, which is like a plastic microphone, on the patient's lower abdomen over the bladder. This is done after the patient has been asked to void, and the probe calculates how much

International Prostate Symptom Score (IPSS) = AUA Symptom Score + QOL question

1. Incomplete emptying
Over the last month, how often have you had a sensation of not emptying your bladder completely after you finished urinating?

2. Frequency
Over the past month, how often have you had the urge to urinate again less than two hours after you finished urinating?

3. Intermittency
Over the past month, how often have you found you stopped and started again several times when you urinated?

4. Urgency
Over the past month, how often have you found it difficult to postpone urination?

5. Weak stream
Over the past month, how often have you had a weak urinary stream?

6. Straining
Over the past month, how often have you had to push or strain to begin urination?

7. Nocturia
Over the past month, how many times did you most typically get up to urinate from the time you went to bed at night until the time you got up in the morning?

Total IPSS Score (max 35):
Interpretation of Symptoms:

(Mild: less than 8; Moderate: 8–19; Severe: 20–35)

Quality of life due to urinary symptoms

If you were to spend the rest of your life with your urinary condition the way it is now, how would you feel about that?

0 points - Not at all 1 point - Less than 1 time in 5 2 points - Less than half the time 3 points - About half the time 4 points - More than half the time 5 points - Almost always	0 points - Not at all 1 point - Less than 1 time in 5 2 points - Less than half the time 3 points - About half the time 4 points - More than half the time 5 points - Almost always
0 points - Not at all 1 point - Less than 1 time in 5 2 points - Less than half the time 3 points - About half the time 4 points - More than half the time 5 points - Almost always	0 points - Not at all 1 point - Less than 1 time in 5 2 points - Less than half the time 3 points - About half the time 4 points - More than half the time 5 points - Almost always
0 points - Not at all 1 point - Less than 1 time in 5 2 points - Less than half the time 3 points - About half the time 4 points - More than half the time 5 points - Almost always	0 points - Not at all 1 point - Less than 1 time in 5 2 points - Less than half the time 3 points - About half the time 4 points - More than half the time 5 points - Almost always

0 points - None
1 point - Once
2 points - Twice
3 points - Three times
4 points - Four times
5 points - Five or more times

Reset

0 points - Delighed
1 point - Pleased
2 points - Mostly satisfied
3 points - Mixed - about equally satisfied and dissatisfied
4 points - Mostly dissatisfied
5 points - Unhappy
6 points - Terrible

Figure 20   International Prostate Symptom Score (IPSS).

urine is left in the bladder. This procedure is totally painless, and a medical assistant, a nurse, or a physician performs this in a physician's office. Bladder scanner/ ultrasound postvoid residual determination is often performed in those men who present with a complaint of the feeling of incomplete bladder emptying and/or those men with urinary incontinence.

Cystoscopy: Cystoscopy means literally *to look into the bladder*. A cystoscope is either a rigid or flexible instrument that has a lens at one end and is connected to a light source. The instrument permits the urologist to look up through the penis and through the prostate and into the bladder. If a rigid cystoscope is used, the patient is placed on his back with his feet in stirrups (**Figure 21**). If a flexible cystoscope is used, the patient is positioned flat on his back with his feet out straight or the supine position. A cystoscopy can be performed with either the patient under general, spinal, or local anesthesia and can

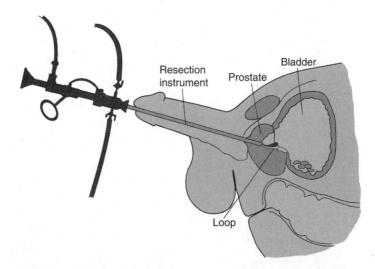

Figure 21   Position for cystoscopy.

Crowley, LV. *An Introduction to Human Disease*. 6th ed. Jones and Bartlett Publishers, LLC. Sudbury, MA, 2004.

be done in either the physician's office or the operating room in the hospital. Not all men with BPH symptoms need cystoscopy. If your doctor notes that you have blood cells in your urine (microscopic hematuria) or you have seen blood in your urine (gross hematuria) you will need a cystoscopy in addition to other tests. In those men with BPH who are considering surgical or minimally invasive treatment the urologist will often perform a cystoscopy before the procedure to make sure that you are a candidate for the procedure and that there are no other abnormalities (bladder stones, bladder tumors, urethral strictures) present. In those individuals who don't respond to medical therapy, a cystoscopy may be indicated.

Urodynamics

A urodynamic study is a test used to assess how well the bladder and urethra are performing their job of storing and releasing urine.

Urodynamic tests can help your doctor assess such symptoms as:

Urinary incontinence

Urinary frequency

Urgency

Problems with starting one's stream (hesitancy)

Painful urination

Incomplete bladder emptying

Recurrent infections

A urodynamic study is comprised of a series of tests. Depending on your symptoms, you many need some or all of the components. Urodynamic studies are often performed in the doctor's office or in a specialized outpatient area.

Little preparation is needed for a urodynamic test. You can eat prior to the test. Your doctor may ask you to come in with a full bladder.

The urodynamic study may start with a uroflow. The uroflow measures the rate of urination in cubic centimeters or milliliters per second (see Question 34). After the uroflow, the cystometrogram (CMG) component of the urodnynamic study is performed. The CMG assesses pressure in the bladder during bladder filling and urinating. After voiding, a specialized catheter is placed into your urethra and passed into your bladder. The catheter is taped in place to prevent if from falling out during the study. Your bladder is emptied and the volume left behind in your bladder after voiding, the postvoid residual (PVR), is recorded. Once the catheter is secured in place and your bladder is emptied, the catheter is connected to a special pressure monitor, a transducer, and to the tubing that supplies the sterile fluid. A separate catheter is placed into your rectum which allows the doctor to measure pressures within your abdomen. The rectal catheter is also connected to a transducer. In order to assess the activity of your pelvic floor muscles skin patch electrodes or small needle electrodes will be placed in the area near your anus. These electrodes measure activity in your pelvic floor muscles, which also surround the urethra. This type of study is called electromyography (EMG). The EMG measures activity in the muscles of the pelvic floor. During the urodynamic study, fluoroscopy (X-ray) may be used to visualize your bladder and urethra during bladder filling and voiding. If X-ray is used during the study it is called video-urodynamics.

After placement of the two catheters and the electrodes, the CMG is started. Sterile fluid is instilled into your bladder at a rate specified by your doctor. A computer screen displays the pressures in your abdomen, your bladder, and the activity of your pelvic floor muscles.

Shortly after starting the study you will be asked to cough or bear down to ensure that the catheters are in the correct position and transducers are working properly. While your bladder is filling with the sterile fluid, your doctor will ask you to indicate when you first feel the urge to void and when you feel a strong urge to void. The volumes in your bladder at each of these times will be recorded.

Normally, during bladder filling the bladder pressure remains very low and the bladder muscle is quiet (stable) until one feels the urge to urinate and decides to void. During voiding, the bladder pressure quickly increases and then promptly decreases as soon as urination is completed. Periodic increases in bladder pressure during the study are referred to as involuntary bladder contractions/detrusor overactivity and may contribute to the symptoms of frequency, urgency, and urge incontinence. The CMG also evaluates **bladder compliance**. Poor compliance, the inability to store urine at low pressures, may cause damage to the kidneys and be a source of urine leakage.

During the study, when you feel a strong urge to urinate, the fluid infusion will be stopped and you will be asked to void. During urination the bladder pressures and the urine flow rate are monitored. These values are then plotted on a nomogram called a **pressure flow study**. This study is particularly helpful in males as it helps determine if there is any significant obstruction

Periodic increases in bladder pressure during the study are referred to as involuntary bladder contractions/ detrusor overactivity and may contribute to the symptoms of frequency, urgency, and urge incontinence.

Bladder compliance

The ability of the bladder to hold increasing amounts of urine without increases in bladder pressure and reflects the elasticity of the bladder.

129

Pressure flow study

A component of a urodynamic study, whereby the bladder pressure is plotted against the urine flow rate. It is useful in determining if obstruction to the outflow of urine is present.

to the outflow of urine. During voiding, the flow rate and electromyelogram (EMG) are assessed. This is helpful in ensuring that there is appropriate relaxation of the pelvic floor muscles prior to voiding and that this relaxation continues throughout voiding.

In some cases, a specialized dye is used to fill your bladder. This allows your doctor to take X-rays periodically during the study to look at your bladder and urethra.

35. What other disorders can mimic BPH?

Other underlying disorders can mimic the symptoms of BPH. A neurogenic bladder, or bladder with impairment of its nerve supply, can cause a patient to void either frequently or infrequently depending on the nature of the neurologic problem. At times, a neurogenic bladder can cause the patient to be unable to urinate or go into urinary retention.

Diabetes mellitus can cause frequent urination, as many patients with diabetes make a greater volume of urine per 24 hours. With long-standing diabetes, bladder damage can occur that results in a decreased ability of the bladder to contract and therefore causes less frequent urination.

A urinary tract infection can cause urinary frequency and burning with urination. A urethral stricture or scar tissue in the urethra from old infections or trauma can cause a decrease in the urinary stream.

The following is a list of additional disorders that may mimic BPH:

- Other causes of bladder outlet obstruction:
- Bladder neck obstruction
- Prostate cancer

- Müllerian duct cysts—congenital abnormalities—if the cysts are large, they may compress the urethra, making it difficult to void
- Urethral stricture—scar tissue in the urethra causing narrowing and resistance to the flow of urine
- Urethral valves—congenital leaflets in the urethra that balloon out, like the sails of a sailboat, when one is urinating and obstruct the outflow of urine

- Impaired detrusor contractility—a bladder that does not contract well
- Overactive bladder—occurs in 40–70% men with bladder outlet obstruction
- Painful bladder syndrome
- Inflammatory and infectious conditions:

  - Cystitis—infection/inflammation of the bladder
  - Carcinoma *in situ* of the bladder—an early cancer in the bladder that may cause the bladder to be overactive
  - Prostatitis (see Question 61)

36. What damage can BPH cause?

Enlargement of the prostate, BPH, increases the resistance to the flow of urine out of the bladder. Thus the bladder needs to work harder to push urine beyond the resistance. In order to accomplish this, the bladder pressures must increase. As a result of this need for increased force there is hypertrophy of the bladder muscle. The increased work that the bladder muscle needs to do to empty the bladder may lead to the development of overactive bladder (Questions 41 and 42). This increased pressure that the bladder needs to generate can be transmitted backwards from the bladder to the kidneys, and in some individuals it may impair the drainage of the kidneys, causing swelling of the kidneys/hydronephrosis and a decrease in kidney function. If the bladder cannot create enough pressure and/or cannot maintain the elevated pressure, then the bladder may not empty completely. This residual urine may put some men at risk for bladder stones, bladder infections (UTI), and if the residual is significant, urinary leakage. Over the course of time, in some males, the bladder decompensates and acute urinary retention may occur, in which the male is unable to urinate. In some men, this is reversible with relief of the obstruction, in others, the bladder never recovers.

37. When does BPH need to be treated?

The need to initiate treatment for BPH is divided into absolute and relative indications. Absolute indications refer to objective medical reasons to intervene. These include impaired renal function because of prostatic obstruction, hydronephrosis or dilation of the ureters and kidneys, recurrent urinary tract infections, bladder stones, and inability to void (urinary retention).

These absolute and relative indications for the treatment of BPH appear in **Table 11**.

The relative indications are for improvement in quality of life if the symptoms of BPH are bothersome and the patient wishes to try to improve them.

Table 11 Indications for BPH Treatment

Absolute	Relative
Impaired renal function	Nocturia
Hydronephrosis	Urinary frequency
Recurrent UTIs	Urinary urgency
Bladder stones	Decreased force of stream
Urinary retention	

Source: Loughlin, P. *100 Questions and Answers About Prostate Disease.* Jones and Bartlett Publishers, LLC, 2007.

38. What are the alpha-blockers?

Alpha-blockers are a class of medications used for the treatment of BPH. Alpha receptors are located within the bladder and the prostate and they modulate tone. Alpha receptors are found in the sympathetic nervous system and throughout the body. They control a variety of physiologic functions, not just voiding.

Alpha receptors respond to norepinephrine and, when norepinephrine binds (attaches) to the alpha receptors, it causes a change in the tone of smooth muscle fibers, increasing the tone. Alpha receptors are found in the smooth muscle of the prostate and the bladder and are important in regulating the prostate tone and the smooth muscle of the bladder.

When alpha receptors in the prostatic smooth muscle are stimulated by norepinephrine, the result is increased tone of the prostatic smooth muscle. A way to think of this is that the prostate squeezes around the urethra and tightens its grip, resulting in increased urethral resistance to urine flow from the bladder. This increased prostatic tone, therefore, can result in the symptoms of bladder outlet obstruction.

Because norepinephrine is the signal that acts on the alpha receptors to cause smooth muscle to contract, if you block part of that signal, you should decrease the muscle contraction. Alpha blockers block the binding of norepinephrine at the alpha adrenergic receptor and thus prevent contraction of the prostatic smooth muscle and thus are useful in treating BPH symptoms.

Over the past decade, an increasing number of alpha blockers have become available on the U.S. market (**Table 12**). They are generally divided into selective and nonselective alpha blockers, depending on which receptors

Table 12   BPH Drugs and Dosing

DRUG	DOSE	Tmax Hrs	Half-Life Hrs	Metab	Contraindications
Alpha-blocker					
Alfuzosin (Uroxatral)	10 mg	8 hrs	10 hrs	Liver metabolism, CYP3A4	Contraindicated in moderate to severe hepatic impairment, should not be used with co administration of potent CYP3A4 inhibitors. Intraoperative Floppy Iris Syndrome has been reported in patients taking uroxatral while undergoing cataract surgery.
Doxazosin (Cardura)	1 mg, 2 mg, 4 mg, 8 mg	2–3 hrs	22 hrs	Liver metabolism mainly by O–demethylation of quinazoline nucleus or hydroxylation of the benzodioxan moiety	Administer with caution if impaired hepatic function. Intraoperative Floppy Iris Syndrome has been reported in patients taking doxazosin while undergoing cataract surgery.
Doxazosin XL (Cardura XL)	4 mg, 8 mg with breakfast	4 mg; 8 ± 3.7 hrs 8 mg; 9 ± 4.7 hrs	15–19 hrs	CYP3A4 primary elimination pathway but also CYP2D6 and CYP2C19	Use with caution in pts with mild or moderate hepatic impairment, not recommended with severe hepatic impairment. Intraoperative Floppy Iris Syndrome has been reported in patients taking doxazosin while undergoing cataract surgery.
Silodosin (Rapaflo)	4 mg and 8 mg capsule, once daily with meal	2.6 ± 0.90 hrs	13.3 ± 8.07 hrs	Glucuronidation, alcohol and aldehyde dehydrogenase, and Cyt P450 pathways	Severe renal impairment. Severe liver impairment. Concomitant admin strong CytP3A4 inhibitors.

Table 12 BPH Drugs and Dosing (*Continued*)

DRUG	DOSE	Tmax Hrs	Half-Life Hrs	Metab	Contraindications
					Silodosin is not recommended in patients taking strong P-gp inhibitors such as cyclosporine. As with other alpha-blockers, individuals taking silodosin should discuss this with opthalmologist prior to undergoing cataract surgery due to risk of Intraoperative Floppy Iris Syndrome.
Tamsulosin (Flomax)	0.4 mg, 0.8 mg	0.4 mg: 4 hrs (fasted), 6 hrs (light breakfast), 0.8 mg: 5.0 hrs (fasted), 7.0 hrs (light breakfast)	0.8 mg: 14.9 ± 3.9	Cyt P450– CYP3A4 and CYP2D6	Use with caution in combination with moderate or strong CYP2D6 or CYP3A4 inhibitors; if pt has a serious or life–threatening sulfa allergy, caution warranted when using tamsulosin. Intraoperative Floppy Iris Syndrome, a complication in cataract surgery, has been reported in patients taking Flomax prior to cataract surgery.
Terazosin (Hytrin)	1 mg, 2 mg, 5 mg, 10 mg capsules, with or without food	1 hr	12 hrs	Extensively metabolized by liver with little parent drug excreted in urine and feces	Contraindicated in those with known sensitivity to terazosin. Same concerns apply regarding use and risk of Intraoperative Floppy Iris Syndrome in patients undergoing cataract surgery.
5-alpha-reductase inbibitors					
Dutasteride (Avodart)	0.5 mg with or without food	2–3 hrs	5 wks at steady state	Liver metabolized by CYP3A4 and CYP3A5	Caution when co administration with potent, chronic CYP3A4 inhibitors.
Finasteride (Proscar)	5 mg	1.8 hrs	6 hrs (3–16 hrs) 8.2 hrs in those ≥ 70 yrs	Liver Metabolized by CYP3A4	Caution with use in those pts with liver function abnormalities.

they block. Selective alpha blockers act primarily on the prostate with fewer systemic effects. Nonselective alpha blockers act both systemically and on the prostate. Both selective and nonselective alpha blockers are effective in treating BPH symptoms. A summary of the currently available alpha blockers and their characteristics appears in Table 12.

The choice of alpha blocker used may depend on your other medical conditions and medications that you are taking, your physician's preference, as well as your insurance plan coverage.

What are the side effects of alpha-blockers?

The side effects of alpha-blocker drugs are primarily caused by blockade of alpha receptor sites outside of the urinary tract. Commonly reported side effects of alpha-blocker drugs include dizziness, headache, asthenia (weakness), postural hypotension (decreased blood pressure with change of body position), rhinitis (inflammation of nasal mucous membranes), and ejaculatory dysfunction. These side effects occur in about 5 to 9% of patients taking the drugs and can be reversed by stopping the drugs.

Combined use of alpha-blockers and PDE-5 inhibitors [sildenafil (Viagra), vardenafil (Levitra), and tadalafil (Cialis)] can lead to significant decreases in blood pressure in some individuals.

Recently, there has been a concern regarding an increased risk of Intraoperative Floppy Iris Syndrome occurring during cataract surgery in individuals taking alpha-blockers. Thus, individuals considering cataract surgery who are on or have taken alpha-blockers should discuss their current/past use of alpha-blockers with the ophthalmologist.

How are they similar and how are they different?

All six of the alpha blockers commonly used today in the United States have been demonstrated to be beneficial in the treatment of BPH symptoms. Phenoxybenzamine (Dibenzyline) and Prazosin (Minipress) are not commonly used anymore because to be effective they have to be taken more than once per day. The medications vary in that some are single dose therapies and others are dose-titratable. Similarly, dosing recommendations with respect to timing in relation to meals varies with the different medications (see Table 12). Although all alpha-blockers have the potential to cause dizziness and postural hypotension, the incidence of these side effects are lower with the selective alpha-blockers such as tamsulosin and silodosin.

All of the alpha blockers have been proven to be more effective than placebo in treating the symptoms of BPH. More selective agents, such as tamsulosin and silodosin are thought to cause less systemic side effects, such as dizziness, hypotension, and fainting.

39. What are the 5-alpha reductase inhibitors?

The 5-alpha reductase inhibitors are a class of medications that inhibit the enzyme 5-alpha reductase. The enzymes 5-alpha reductase are present in two isoforms: type 1 and type 2. Type 1 is found predominantly in extraprostatic tissues such as the skin and liver, although it is also found in the prostate. Type 2 is found predominantly in the prostate. The type 2 5-alpha reductase enzyme in the prostate is responsible for converting testosterone to its active form in the prostate, dihydrotestosterone. Dihydrotestosterone mediates secondary sexual characteristics, including prostate growth (**Figure 22**).

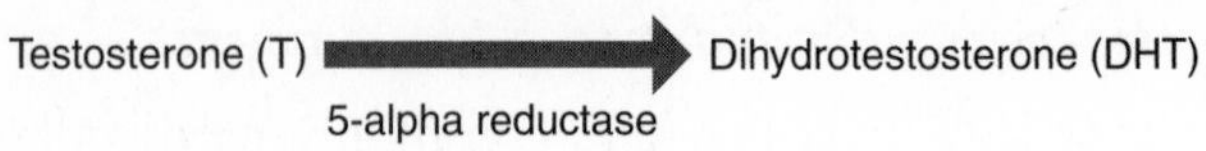

Testosterone (T) ➡️ Dihydrotestosterone (DHT)
5-alpha reductase

Figure 22   Action of 5-alpha reductase.

Two drugs have been developed that inhibit 5-alpha reductase. The first is finasteride or Proscar, which is a type 2 or selective 5-alpha reductase inhibitor. The second is dutasteride or Avodart, which is a type 1 and type 2 or nonselective 5-alpha reductase inhibitor. (Table 12) Finasteride has been shown to reduce serum DHT levels by 70%, whereas dutasteride has been shown to reduce serum DHT by 90%. It is not yet known whether that difference in DHT suppression translates into greater efficacy for the patient. 5-alpha reductase inhibitors work best in men with noticeable enlargement of the prostate.

What are the side effects of 5-alpha reductase inhibitors?

Side effects found in the first year of 5-alpha reductase inhibitor use include: decreased sexual drive (libido), increased ejaculatory dysfunction (such as smaller amount of semen ejaculated), difficulty getting an erection, breast tenderness or enlargement. One large study demonstrated that after a year of treatment, finasteride resulted in the same level of decreased sex drive and inability to get an erection as placebo. Ejaculatory dysfunction was higher with finasteride than with placebo.

What are the results of BPH treatment using 5-alpha reductase inhibitor drugs?

As mentioned previously, finasteride (Proscar) and dutasteride (Avodart) are the two 5-alpha reductase inhibitors that are currently available in the United States. Both of these drugs require 3 to 6 months to see clinical beneficial effects. The Finasteride Study Group showed improvement in peak flow rates and symptom scores as well as a decrease in prostate volume. At 1 year, patients on 5 milligrams of finasteride had a 22% improvement in peak flow rates and a 21% decrease in symptom scores. In addition, they exhibited a 19% decrease in their prostate volume.

A recent report looking at cohort of patients treated with dutasteride showed similar improvement in urinary flow rates, a decrease in symptom scores, and a reduction in prostate volume.

What effects do 5-alpha reductase inhibitor drugs have on PSA levels?

5-alpha reductase inhibitor drugs block the conversion of testosterone to DHT, which results in shrinkage of the prostate or a decrease in prostate volume. Because prostate cells make PSA, it is reasonable to assume that as the prostate gets smaller, the PSA level will decline. This is in fact what happens; however, it takes 3 to 6 months for a significant volume decrease to occur, and thus, the PSA decline is gradual. Nonetheless, by about 6 months after starting a 5-alpha reductase inhibitor, the total PSA level is about half of the baseline value. The free fraction of PSA is not changed by treatment with 5-alpha reductase inhibitors. In patients who have been on 5-alpha reductase inhibitors for longer than 3–6 months, the PSA should remain stable and significant increases in the PSA would be worrisome for prostate cancer.

In patients who have been on 5-alpha reductase inhibitors for longer than 3–6 months, the PSA should remain stable and significant increases in the PSA would be worrisome for prostate cancer.

Do the 5-alpha reductase inhibitors have an effect on the risk of developing prostate cancer?

A recent study called the "Prostate Cancer Prevention Trial" (PCPT) demonstrated that finasteride (Proscar) at a dose of 5mg/day decreases the likelihood of developing prostate cancer by 26% when compared to placebo (candy pill). In addition, finasteride decreased the risk of high grade PIN (which may be a precursor of prostate cancer) by about the same rate. In this study, finasteride lowered the PSA by 50% after 2 months of treatment.

"Asymptomatic men with a PSA ≤ 3.0 ng/ml who are regularly screened with PSA or who are anticipating undergoing annual PSA screening for early detection of prostate cancer may benefit from a discussion of both the benefits of 5-alpha reductase inhibitors for 7 years for the prevention of prostate cancer and the potential risks (2–4% increase in reported erectile dysfunction and gynecomastia (enlarged and/or painful breasts), and decrease in ejaculate volume in those receiving finasteride in the study compared to those receiving placebo)."

www.auanet.org/content/guidelines-and-quality-care/clinical-guidelines/main-reports/pcredinh.pdf.

Results of the "Reduction by Dutasteride of Prostate Cancer" (REDUCE) trial showed that the 5-alpha reductase inhibitor dutasteride at doses of 0.5 mg/day decreased the relative risk of prostate cancer by 23% compared to placebo. Furthermore, the risk was markedly decreased in the number of high-grade tumors, with no absolute increase in incidence compared to placebo.

40. Can alpha-blocker drugs and 5-alpha reductase drugs be used together?

The short answer to this question is yes. For several years, many urologists used these drugs together with the rationale that because their mechanisms of action were different, their benefits might be additive; however, there was no objective proof that this really was so. In 2003, the MTOPS (The Medical Therapy of Prostate Symptoms) study was published in the *New England Journal of Medicine* (2003;349). It looked at whether a combination of both kinds of drugs was better than either drug alone.

This study was a double-blind (neither the investigator or study participants knew who received drug(s) or placebo) trial that involved more than 3,000 men who were followed for an average of 4.5 years. The men were divided into four groups: placebo (control group), doxazosin (an alpha blocker) alone, finasteride alone, and doxazosin and finasteride together. These four groups of patients were then followed for signs of progression of BPH. Progression was defined as an increase of urinary symptoms, as measured by the American Urological Association symptom score, acute urinary retention, urinary incontinence, renal insufficiency, or recurrent urinary tract infections. The risk reduction of signs of progression of BPH was 39% with doxazosin, 34% with finasteride, and 66% with combination therapy.

MTOPS proved that the two classes of drugs used together were superior compared with either type of drug alone; however, the practical issue is cost. Obviously, two drugs cost more than one. Therefore, in most cases, the physician will start treatment with one class of drug or the other and add the second drug only if the response to the first drug alone is not satisfactory.

41. What are LUTs?

Lower urinary tract symptoms is a term used to apply to both storage and emptying symptoms. In the field of urology, this term has replaced *BPH sx*. BPH symptoms are part of the voiding phase lower urinary tract symptoms (LUTs).

LUTs include storage and voiding symptoms. Storage (overactive bladder) symptoms include urinary frequency (voiding eight or more times per day), urinary urgency (a sudden compelling desire to void that is difficult to defer), nocturia, and urgency urinary incontinence.

Voiding symptoms include decreased force of stream, hesitancy, straining to void, postterminal dribbling, and intermittency of the urine stream.

A significant number of men presenting with voiding symptoms suggestive of underlying benign prostatic hypertrophy will also have storage symptoms, thus the term LUTs would be more appropriate in these individuals. Medical therapy designed to treat the voiding phase symptoms may or may not lead to improvement in the storage symptoms. Men may have underlying overactive bladder in addition to BPH and studies have demonstrated that with relief of the outflow obstruction associated with BPH there may be improvement in the overactive bladder symptoms. However, in men undergoing transurethral prostatectomy for BPH, 30% of men after relief of their bladder outlet obstruction, had persistent overactive bladder symptoms.

42. What happens if storage (overactive bladder) symptoms persist after successful treatment of the voiding symptoms?

In males with LUTs in whom the voiding (BPH) symptoms have been successfully treated, but whose overactive bladder symptoms persist, a trial of antimuscarinic therapy can be tried if there is no contraindication to the use of antimuscarinic agents. Your doctor will want to make sure that you are emptying your bladder well before using an antimuscarinic. There are a variety of antimuscarinic agents available (**Table 13**). They all are effective in decreasing urinary frequency, urgency, and urgency

Table 13   Antimuscarinic Dosing, Pharmacokinetics, and Metabolism

Medication	Dose	Half-life, hrs	Time to Peak (hr)	Metabolism
OXYBUTYNIN				
Oxybutynin IR (Ditropan)	2.5 to 5 mg BID to TID	2–3 hrs	<1	Liver
Oxybutynin ER (Ditropan XL)	5–30 mg/day	12–13 hrs	3–6	Liver
Oxybutynin transdermal patch (Oxytrol)	36 mg patch delivers 3.9 mg/day. Apply twice a week.	7–8	10–48	Liver
Oxybutynin suspension	5 mg TID	4 hrs	0.5 to 1.4	Liver
Oxybutynin chloride gel (Gelnique 10%)	1 gram unit dose of 10 mg/g/day (1.14 ml).	64 hrs at steady state	Steady-state concentrations achieved within 7 days of steady dosing.	Liver
TOLTERODINE				
Tolterodine IR (Detrol IR)	1–2 mg BID	2–4 hrs	1–2	Liver
Tolterodine LA (Detrol LA)	2–4 mg QD	7–18 hrs	2–6	Liver
TROSPIUM CHLORIDE				
Trospium Chloride IR (Sanctura)	20 mg BID 1 hour before meals	18 hrs	5–6	Ester hydrolysis Renal excretion
Trospium Chloride XR (Sanctura XR)	60 mg QD 1 hr before breakfast	36 hrs	5	Ester hydrolysis Renal excretion
Fesoterodine (Toviaz)	4–8 mg QD	7–8 hrs	5	Ester hydrolysis Liver Renal excretion
Solifenacin (Vesicare)	5–10 mg QD	45–68 hrs	3–8	Liver
Darifenacin (Enablex)	7.5–15 mg QD	7–20 hrs	5–8	Liver

incontinence episodes. The most common side effects of the antimuscarinics are dry mouth and constipation. Rarely, some may affect cognition (memory and learning) or cause visual disturbances. These medications are contraindicated in individuals who have a history of narrow angle (the less common type of glaucoma) glaucoma, gastric (stomach) emptying problems, and urinary retention. If you have any concerns regarding potential side effects or interactions with any of your current medications it is important to talk to your doctor.

43. What is the role of herbal therapy in BPH treatment?

This question is difficult to answer. Herbs are considered as food additives and not drugs and, as such, are not regulated by the FDA. The production and marketing of herbs are essentially unregulated. Therefore, few randomized studies evaluate the efficacy of herbal therapy in the treatment of BPH.

Phytotherapy, more commonly known as herbal therapy, has become increasingly popular in the treatment of BPH. About 30 herbal compounds have been used to treat prostatic urinary symptoms. The most popular of these is saw palmetto, which is the extract of the dried ripe fruit from the American dwarf saw palmetto plant, *Serenoa repens*.

Until recently, the efficacy of saw palmetto was unknown. A 2006 study in the *New England Journal of Medicine* (2006;354:557–566), however, demonstrated that there was no significant difference between saw palmetto and placebo as measured by symptom scores or urinary flow rates. Unless subsequent reports refute this well-done study, it would seem that saw palmetto has no documented benefit in the treatment of BPH.

44. What happens if medical therapy fails or one cannot tolerate the adverse effects of medical therapy?

For men who fail or cannot tolerate medical therapy there are a variety of additional options available for treatment of BPH. These options vary from minimally invasive procedures to open surgical procedures. The choice of procedure will be determined by your overall health status, the size of your prostate, the presence or absence of other problems, such as bladder stones, your preference, and your urologist's recommendations. Surgical interventions include open prostatectomy, transurethral prostatectomy, transurethral incision of the prostate, and various laser treatments of the prostate. Minimally invasive approaches to treatment of BPH include microwave therapy, transurethral needle ablation (TUNA), radiofrequency ablation of the prostate, and placement of prostatic stents. In those individuals in retention, in whom urodynamic studies have demonstrated poor bladder function, an indwelling foley catheter, suprapubic catheter, or clean intermittent catheterization are options.

45. What is an open prostatectomy?

An open prostatectomy is the removal of the obstructing portion of a benign prostate through a surgical incision. Open prostatectomies are usually reserved for large prostates that weigh more than 100 grams. The open prostatectomy allows for the greatest amount of prostate tissue to be removed, but the morbidity is greater than less invasive options because it is an open surgical procedure.

The most common approach to performing an open prostatectomy is through a lower abdominal incision that extends from the symphysis pubis to the umbilicus (belly button) (**Figure 23**).

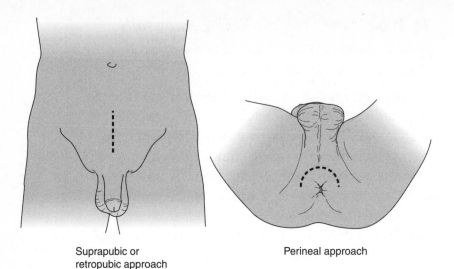

Suprapubic or
retropubic approach

Perineal approach

Figure 23   Types of surgical incisions for simple prostatectomy: suprapubic or retropubic approach and perineal approach.

After the surgeon enters the abdomen through this incision, he or she has two surgical choices. The first is to make an incision in the front wall of the bladder to approach the prostate. This is called a suprapubic prostatectomy. After the surgeon has entered the bladder, he or she can enucleate, or shell out, the center of the prostate with his or her index finger. After the inner portion of the prostate is enucleated, stitches are placed in the prostatic fossa (the shell of prostate that is left). Postoperatively, the patient is left with a urethral catheter coming out of his penis and a suprapubic catheter coming out of the lower abdomen. A patient is usually in the hospital 3 or 4 days after a suprapubic prostatectomy.

A retropubic simple prostatectomy is similar to a suprapubic simple prostatectomy as it is also performed through a lower abdominal incision. When performing a retropubic simple prostatectomy, however, the urologist does not open the bladder but instead makes an incision through the prostate capsule. As is done with a suprapubic prostatectomy, the inner portion of the prostate is enucleated. Because the bladder is not opened, it is not necessary to leave a suprapubic tube postoperatively, but a urethral catheter is left in place. Like a suprapubic simple prostatectomy, the patient is usually in the hospital 3 or 4 days postoperatively. The retropubic approach tends to be associated with less bladder irritation after the procedure since the bladder itself is not opened.

In addition to the abdominal approaches described previously here, a benign prostate can be surgically approached via the perineum (Figure 23). When this approach is used, the perineal skin incision is used to expose the prostate; then an incision is made in the prostatic capsule, and the prostate is enucleated, similar to a simple retropubic prostatectomy. A urethral catheter is left postoperatively, and the patient is usually in the hospital 1 to 2 days.

46. What is a transurethral prostatectomy (TURP)?

A transurethral prostatectomy (TURP) is an operation designed to remove the prostate through the urethra; no external incision is made. A TURP is performed using a resectoscope, which scrapes out the center of the prostate by using an electrical current to cut out the tissue with a loop. This procedure is ideal for men with small to moderate size prostate glands. It is difficult to perform in men with extremely large prostates, i.e. those 100 grams or larger, due to the duration of time that it takes to resect the prostate tissue and the risks incurred with the lengthy resection. Lengthy resections pose the risk of absorbing too much of the irrigation fluid and lowering the salt level in the blood stream (hyponatremia) In severe cases, hyponatremia can cause neurologic symptoms, including seizures. Fortunately, these complications occur vary rarely. TURPs are usually limited to prostate glands of 100 grams or smaller.

After the TURP has been completed, a urethral catheter is left to enable irrigation of the bladder with fluid to prevent blood clots from forming in the bladder, typically for 1 to 2 days. After that period of time, the catheter is removed, and the patient is given a voiding trial. Sometimes, a patient will have troubles urinating right after a TURP and if this is the case, then the catheter will be replaced and left in place for about a week and another trial of voiding will be performed.

47. What is a transurethral incision of the prostate (TUIP)?

A transurethral incision of the prostate (TUIP) is exactly that: an incision rather than a resection of the prostate. Using a special knife-like instrument, a Colling's knife that is placed through the same resectoscope sheath used for TURPs two incisions are made at 5 o'clock and 7 o'clock through the bladder neck and prostate to the verumontanum where the ejaculatory ducts exit.

A TUIP is a quicker, easier procedure than a TURP. TUIPs tend to be used in younger men with smaller prostate glands. The incidence of retrograde ejaculation after TURP ranges from 50 to 95%, whereas the incidence is from 0 to 37% with TUIP. In properly selected patients, those with small glands, the rate of symptom relief with TUIP approaches that of TURP.

48. What is electrovaporization of the prostate?

Electrovaporization of the prostate (TUVP) is, similar to a TURP. Rather than a resecting loop, the urologist uses a roller ball to heat and desiccate the prostate instead of actually resecting tissue (**Figure 24**).

Electrovaporization of the prostate has been used in patients with a history of bleeding disorders or in cases in which it is desired to minimize blood loss. Electrovaporization of the prostate tends to be used in patients with small- and medium-sized glands. Like TUIP, in properly selected patients, it is an alternative to TURP.

49. What are the side effects of surgical treatment (TURP) of BPH?

The side effects associated with TURP can be divided into intraoperative and postoperative complications. A TURP is performed under either spinal or general anesthesia,

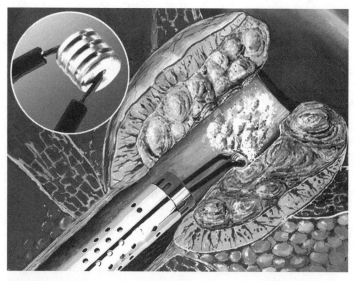

Figure 24   Electovaporization of the prostate using a TURP VaporTrode™.

Courtesy of Gyrus ACMI, Southborough, MA

and the usual complications that are associated with these forms of anesthesia can occur during a TURP. The introduction of either spinal or general anesthesia can result in hypotension or a drop in blood pressure.

Bleeding can occur with a TURP, and it is correlated with the size of the prostate and the duration of the operation; however, it should be emphasized that significant bleeding is uncommon when an experienced urologist performs the TURP.

Extravasation or perforation of the prostate can occur during a TURP. This causes some of the irrigation fluid used during a TURP to extravasate, or leak outside the prostate. If the patient is awake under spinal anesthesia, this can result in nausea, vomiting, or abdominal pain. Most often, this complication can be managed by cessation of the operation and urethral catheter drainage. As with bleeding, extravasation in the hands of an experienced resectionist is uncommon.

The most dramatic complication that occurs intraoperatively or in the immediate postoperative period is TUR syndrome. TUR syndrome occurs when there is too much absorption of the irrigation fluid and resultant lowering of the salt level in the blood, hyponatremia. The manifestations of the TUR syndrome include nausea, vomiting, brachycardia or slow heart rate, and visual disturbances.

The treatment of the TUR syndrome is principally diuretic medications, which help the patient urinate out the excess fluid that has been absorbed. Some urologists will also give high concentration saline or high-concentration sodium solutions to increase the serum sodium. In most circumstances, the TUR syndrome can be corrected in the immediate postoperative period.

Recent studies report that blood transfusions are required in about 4% of the patients who undergo the procedure. Because the apex of the prostate is near the external urinary sphincter, incontinence is a potential complication. Fortunately, the risk of urinary incontinence after a TURP has been estimated to be about 1%. Erectile dysfunction or impotence can occur after a TURP. It is theorized that some of the electrical current from the resectoscope loupe scatters beyond the prostate capsule and injures the nerves. Other complications include urethral stricture and urinary tract infection.

50. What are the results of TURP for BPH?

The TURP is a common surgical procedure that urologists have performed for decades. It is the gold standard to which other minimally invasive surgical treatments are compared. Subjective and objective success rates with TURP are reported to be 85–90%. The long-term results of a TURP are well established, with durable objective improvements demonstrated 10 years post-procedure.

51. What is minimally invasive surgical treatment of BPH?

Even though open prostatectomy and TURP, TUIP, and TUVP are commonly performed, reliable operations, urologists have sought procedures that are less invasive and easier on the patients. These procedures have become known as minimally invasive surgical treatment (MIST) of BPH. These MIST techniques include VaporTrode procedure, laser procedures, hyperthermia and thermotherapy, radiofrequency ablation, balloon dilation of the prostate, urethral stents, and high-intensity focused ultrasound.

The VaporTrode (CIRCON/ACMI) uses high electrical energy transmitted through a grooved rollerball that is run over the area of prostate to be treated. VaporTrode prostectomy uses the same instrumentation as a TURP, but instead of a resecting loop, the VaporTrode device is used. This vaporizes the prostate tissue. The advantage of VaporTrode is that there is less bleeding. A long-term study comparing subjective and objective outcomes of TURP and VaporTrode demonstrated similar subjective outcomes for both with an average of 10 years of follow-up, with slightly better objective outcomes with TURP.

52. What is laser therapy of the prostate?

Since the 1980s, several generations of lasers have been used to treat obstructive prostate symptoms. LASER is an acronym for light-amplification stimulated emission resonance. In practical terms, this means that the light energy is very focused and allows powerful and precise application of the light energy to tissue.

The potential advantages of laser therapy include minimal bleeding, avoidance of TUR syndrome, less retrograde ejaculation, the ability to treat patients on blood thinners (such as Warfarin [Coumadin] and aspirin), and the potential to treat patients on an outpatient basis.

53. What types of laser therapy are available?

A variety of laser therapies are available. Not every urologist or every hospital has access to every laser available on the market. The following are some of the laser therapies used to treat BPH:

Interstitial laser coagulation: This procedure is performed under local anesthesia on an outpatient basis. The Indigo Laser Optic Treatment system is used with a cystoscope through which a fiberoptic probe is inserted into the prostate. The prostate is heated via the probe for about 3 minutes and this coagulates the obstructing prostatic tissue. The procedure can be repeated in different areas of the prostate. The procedure takes about 30 to 60 minutes to perform. After the procedure is performed an indwelling foley catheter is placed which is usually removed in a few days. It is not uncommon to see some blood in the urine after the procedure, which usually clears in a week. Rarely, erectile dysfunction, retrograde ejaculation, and incontinence can occur.

Photoselective vaporization of the prostate (PVP): This procedure uses a special high-energy laser (e.g., GreenLight PVP™ Laser) to vaporize excess prostate tissue and seal the treated area (**Figures 25a** and **b**). The procedure is performed on an outpatient basis in a hospital or surgical center and may be performed under local, spinal, or general anesthesia. The procedure takes about 30 minutes to perform, depending on the size of the prostate, and patients are usually discharged within a few hours. As with interstitial laser coagulation, the procedure is performed via a cystoscope. Many patients do not require a catheter after PVP, and those who do typically are catheterized for less than 24 hours.

HoLAP (holmium laser ablation of the prostate): This procedure involves using a laser to vaporize obstructive prostatic tissue. The decision whether to use HoLAP or HoLEP (holmium enucleation of the prostate) is based primarily on the size of the prostate. Ablation usually is performed when the prostate is smaller than 60 cc (cubic centimeters).

HoLAP offers many of the same advantages as HoLEP when compared to traditional surgery (e.g., TURP). These potential benefits include a shorter hospital stay, less bleeding, and shorter catheterization and recovery times. Patients who undergo HoLAP usually do not

153

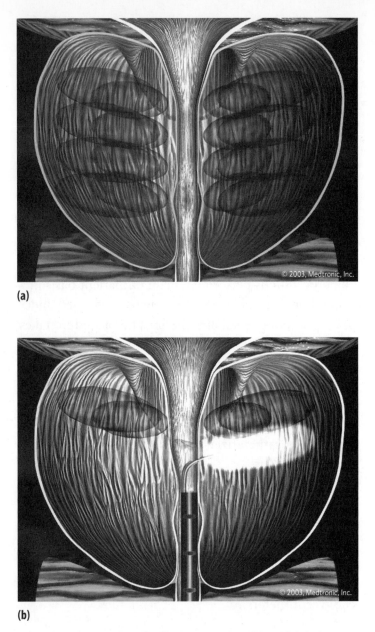

(a)

(b)

Figure 25   (a) Formation of lesions in the prostate. (b) Multiple lesions formed in the prostate.

Courtesy of Medtronic, Inc. © Copyright 2003.

require overnight hospitalization and in most cases, the catheter is removed the same day or the morning following the procedure.

54. What are the results of laser therapy?

Laser therapy for BPH is a relatively new technique, thus series with large numbers of patients followed over an extended period of time are limited. In a Cochrane review of 20 studies involving 1,898 patients, laser techniques were found to be useful and relatively safe alternatives to TURP. Improvements in LUTs and urine flow rate were noted to be slightly better in the TURP group, though laser procedures had fewer side effects and required shorter hospitalization. In one recent study comparing TURP to contact laser treatment, comparable subjective improvements with an average follow-up of 10 years postprocedure, however, only with patients treated with TURP showed durable objective improvements at an average follow-up of 10 years. As with any procedure, it is important to ask your doctor about his/her personal results with performing the procedure.

55. What is microwave therapy of the prostate?

Microwave energy has been used to treat BPH using both transrectal and transurethral approaches, but most modern machines use the transurethral route. Current machines deliver microwave energy to the prostate via a transurethral catheter, and a transrectal balloon monitors rectal temperature simultaneously.

The treatment is delivered under local anesthesia on an outpatient basis and typically takes about one-half hour. The patient will go home with an indwelling urethral catheter for a period of days at the discretion of the urologist.

56. What are the results of microwave therapy?

Results after microwave therapy are either subjective and objective. Subjective results use patient symptoms score sheets where the patients record their perception of their voiding characteristics. Objective results, such as measurements of peak urinary flow rates and post void residual volumes, are measured by the physician. Several studies have shown improvement in both subjective and objective measurement following microwave therapy. This technology is still relatively new, and long-term data are lacking. No one yet knows whether these promising early results are durable.

In a Cochrane review, microwave therapy was found to be a relatively safe and effective treatment option for BPH. Microwave therapy has fewer, as well as less severe, side effects than TURP. TURP produced greater improvement in urinary symptoms and fewer men required retreatment for symptomatic BPH.

57. What is radiofrequency therapy of the prostate and the results of radiofrequency therapy?

This technique involves placing interstitial radiofrequency needles through the urethra into the lateral prostatic lobes to cause coagulation necrosis.

Radiofrequency treatment of BPH is commonly referred to as TUNA—transurethral needle ablation of the prostate. This technique involves placing interstitial radiofrequency needles through the urethra into the lateral prostatic lobes to cause coagulation necrosis. The tissue is heated to 110°C at a radiofrequency power of 490 KHz for 4 minutes per lesion. The number of times the needles are placed into the prostatic lobes is at the discretion of the urologist based on the size of the prostate gland.

The TUNA device and generator are shown in **Figures 26** and **27**. Two needles that are at 60 degree angles to each other are deployed into the prostatic tissues by piercing the prostatic urethra. Each treatment with the needles treats prostate tissue about 1 cm in diameter.

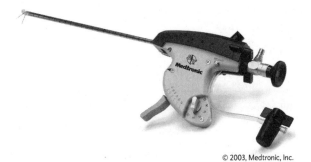

© 2003, Medtronic, Inc.

Figure 26   Precision™ Plus Hand Piece.

Courtesy of Medtronic, Inc. © Copyright 2003.

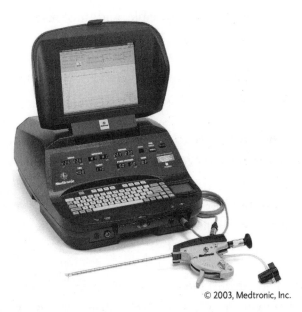

© 2003, Medtronic, Inc.

Figure 27   Precision™ Plus System (computer and hand piece).

Couresty of Medtronic, Inc © Copyright 2003.

Table 14   TUNA Combined Statistics

	Month Post Treatment	Number Patients	Preoperative	Postoperative	Percent Change
IPSS decrease	0	254	22		
Patient rerated	3	213		9	59
Symptom scores	6	150		8	64
	12	29			
Qmax increase	0	254	8 ml/second		
Maximum	3	219		13	63
Urinary flowrate	6	136		13	63
	12	35		14	75

Source: Loughlin, P. *100 Questions and Answers About Prostate Disease.* Jones and Bartlett Publishers, LLC, 2007.

TUNA of the prostate uses radiofrequency energy to treat the patient. As with most of the other MIST results, few long-term data are available, and thus, results must be viewed with caution.

Table 14 contains combined TUNA results using both subjective and objective criteria.

58. What are prostatic stents? What are the results with prostatic stents?

Prostatic stents are devices that are placed transurethrally and expand to keep the prostatic urethra open. In many ways, they are similar to the coronary artery stents that have gained wide notoriety.

Prostatic stents are most commonly used in older men who are in urinary retention requiring an indwelling urethral catheter and who are not candidates for any type of invasive therapy. After the stents have been in place for a few months, the mucosa or lining of the urethra grows through them, and they no longer can be seen cystoscopically.

As mentioned, in properly selected patients, prostatic stents can be very useful. The results of one specific type of prostatic stent called the UROLUME appear in **Table 15**.

Table 15 36-Month Follow-up North American Urolume Study

	Month Post Treatment	Number Patients	Preoperative	Percent Postoperative	Percent Change
Nonretention Cohort					
SS (Madsen) decrease	0	95	14		
Symptom score	36	95		5	65
Qmax increase	0	95	9 ml/second		
Maximum urinary flow rate	36	95		15	67
PVR decrease	0	95	89 ml		
Postroid residual	36	95		54	40
Retention Cohort					
SS (Madsen)	36	31	Retention	5	
Qmax	36	31	Retention	11 ml/second	
PVR	36	31	Retention	46 ml	

Source: Loughlin, P. *100 Questions and Answers About Prostate Disease.* Jones and Bartlett Publishers, LLC, 2007.

59. What is the role of a permanent indwelling urethral catheter in the treatment of BPH?

Some patients with prostatic obstruction and a weak bladder will not be able to void, regardless of what type of surgical intervention is employed. Some of these patients elect to be managed with an indwelling urethral catheter. The main drawback to an indwelling catheter is infection and irritation. In addition, sometimes the catheter can become plugged with blood or debris and needs to be changed emergently. Most patients with an indwelling urethral catheter have it changed by a visiting nurse at home or in the emergency room or their doctor's office at 1- to 2-month intervals.

An alternative to an indwelling urethral catheter is a suprapubic tube. A suprapubic tube can be placed percutaneously into the bladder through the lower abdominal wall. Many patients find a suprapubic tube more comfortable and easier to manage than a urethral catheter. Either the suprapubic tube or urethral catheter is connected to a drainage bag, which can be worn on the leg or hung on the side of a bed. A suprapubic tube is typically changed by a nurse or physician as is the urethral catheter every 1 to 2 months.

60. What is the role of a clean intermittent catheterization in the treatment of BPH?

In individuals with BPH who fail to respond to medical therapy, who are not candidates for surgical therapy, and in whom bladder emptying is a problem, clean intermittent catheterization is an alternative to an indwelling foley catheter. If a patient has mobility of his hands and is motivated, he can be easily taught how to perform clean intermittent catheterization. With clean intermittent catheterization, one places a clean, not sterile catheter, into the urethra and passes the catheter into the bladder to drain urine from the bladder. This procedure is performed anywhere from 3 to 6 times per day, depending on how much urine is drained with each catheterization. The catheters are cleaned in between each catheterization and the same catheter may be used for up to a month before changing to a new catheter. If an individual is unable or unwilling to perform self-catheterization, a family member or caregiver can be taught how to perform clean intermittent catheterization.

61. What is prostatitis?

Prostatitis refers to an inflammation of the prostate gland that can be manifested in a variety of ways. Symptoms of acute bacterial prostatitis include urinary frequency, urgency dysuria or painful urination, nocturia, perineal pain, low back pain, fever, and/or chills. Some men with acute bacterial prostatitis may present with inability to urinate and will require a catheter or suprapubic tube placement until the inflammation and pain have resolved. Some men with acute prostatitis may develop a prostatic abscess that will require drainage. Chronic bacterial prostatitis may present in a similar manner, but men are typically less toxic in appearance.

Prostatitis normally does not occur in children or adolescents, but can occur in adult men of any age. The diagnosis can be elusive and treatment is often empiric.

What types of prostatitis are there?

The National Institutes of Health (NIH) has recently defined the different prostatitis syndromes:

Prostatitis syndromes: NIH classification

I. Acute bacterial prostatitis
II. Chronic bacterial prostatitis

III. Chronic prostatitis/chronic pelvic pain syndrome (CPPS)

A. Inflammatory

B. Noninflammatory

Asymptomatic inflammatory prostatitis

Acute bacterial prostatitis is usually a sudden illness with irritative urinary symptoms and can be associated with fever. Urinary and/or prostatic secretions are often positive for bacteria. Some patients with acute prostatitis will have a transient elevation of their PSA. A PSA should not be done during an episode of acute prostatitis. If a PSA is inadvertently drawn during an episode of acute prostatitis and comes back elevated, a repeat PSA should be obtained after a course of antibiotics has been administered. Chronic bacterial prostatitis tends to be a more indolent condition. Irritative urinary symptoms are typical; however, fever is rare, and positive cultures are uncommon.

62. How is prostatitis diagnosed?

The patient's clinical history, general appearance, and urinalysis are often suggestive of acute bacterial prostatitis. A urine culture is commonly positive for a urinary tract infection. A digital rectal examination will usually identify a very tender prostate. In rare cases, fluctuance may be palpable in the prostate, if there is a prostatic abscess. In men who appear toxic or who fail to improve with antibiotic therapy, a transrectal ultrasound may be obtained to rule out a prostatic abscess. An assessment of postvoid residual is performed. The classic diagnostic maneuver for bacterial prostatitis is the three-glass test. The patient is asked to void and collect his first 10 ml of urine. This is sent for culture and is known as VB1. Then the patient is asked to collect a midstream urine sample after he voids about 200 ml. This urine sample is sent for culture and is known as VB2. Then the urologist performs a digital rectal exam and massages the patient's prostate in an attempt to express prostatic secretions (EPS) into a sterile container. A prostatic massage is not always successful in producing sufficient secretions, and for some men, it can be quite uncomfortable. After the prostatic massage, the patient is asked to void again into a container, referred to as VB3, and this sample is sent for culture. If there is an increase in the number of bacterial colonies seen in either EPS or VB3, a diagnosis of bacterial prostatitis is made, and treatment is based on the antibiotic sensitivities of the organisms that were isolated. If there are no bacteria present, but white blood cells are present in the VB3 collection, it is suggestive of nonbacterial inflammatory prostatitis.

63. How is prostatitis treated?

The treatment of bacterial prostatitis is with antibiotics. Patients with acute bacterial prostatitis may require a short stay in the hospital for intravenous antibiotics and then continue on antibiotics for 2 to 4 weeks. Men with chronic bacterial prostatitis may require a longer course of antibiotics. In those men with recurrent chronic bacterial prostatitis, the doctor may prescribe a low dose of antibioctics for 6 months to prevent recurrent infections. Often bacterial prostatitis is treated with a class of antibiotics called quinolones (for example, ciprofloxacin, norfloxacin, ofloxacin). For men who are allergic to quinolones alternative antibiotics may be used, depending on the sensitivity results of the urine culture. Such alternative antibiotics include doxycycline, minocycline, trimethoprim-sulfamethoxazole, and trimethoprim.

If there is an increase in the number of bacterial colonies seen in either EPS or VB3, a diagnosis of bacterial prostatitis is made, and treatment is based on the antibiotic sensitivities of the organisms that were isolated.

Because nonbacterial prostatitis is also recognized and is often thought to be caused by *Chlamydia trachomatis*, some urologists will give the patient a course of doxycycline, an antibiotic that covers Chlamydia particularly well.

PART THREE

Erectile Dysfunction (ED)

What is erectile dysfunction and how common is it?

What are the current treatment options available for erectile dysfunction?

Is there a role for sex therapy and counseling in the treatment of erectile dysfunction?

More . . .

64. How do erections normally occur?

In order to understand how an erection occurs, one must first learn a little about the anatomy of the penis. The penis may look like one simple tube, but it is actually comprised of three cylinders. There are two on the top of the penis called the corpora cavernosa (a Latin phrase meaning, roughly, "bodies composed of hollows or caves") and one on the underside of the penis, the corpus spongiosum ("sponge-like body") (**Figure 28**). The tip of the penis, called the glans, is part of the corpus spongiosum. The corpora cavernosa are surrounded by a fibroelastic layer of tissue, the tunica albuginea (literally, "white coat," referring to fact that the tunica albuginea is a thick white membrane wrapped around the

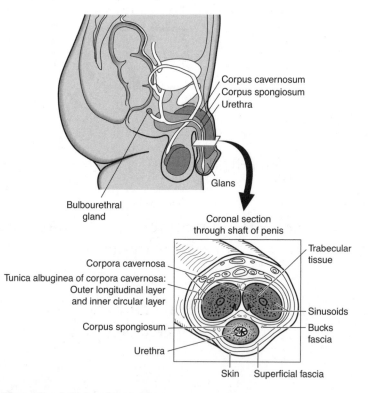

Figure 28   Anatomy of the penis.

Reprinted with permission from *Br J Urol Intl* 2001; 88(Suppl 3):3–10.

corpora cavernosa like a cloak). The two corpora cavernosa contain numerous compartments that are filled with blood during sexual excitement, which is what makes the penis become erect. The corpus spongiosum contains the urethra, the tube that one urinates through, and it is not involved in the erectile process.

The two corpora cavernosa and the corpus spongiosum each have an **artery** that supplies it. The artery to each corpus cavernosum runs through its center (**Figure 29**). The two corpora cavernosa communicate in the middle of the penis, thus allowing blood from one corpus cavernosum to flow into the other. The **veins** that drain the penis are also different for the corpus spongiosum and the corpora cavernosa. The veins that drain the corpora cavernosa, unlike the arteries, run along the outer edge of the corpora cavernosa, just underneath the tunica albuginea (Figure 29).

The reason why these veins and arteries are important is that when a man becomes aroused, his brain and the

Artery

A blood vessel that carries oxygenated blood from the heart to other parts of the body.

Vein

A blood vessel in the body that carries deoxygenated blood from the tissues back to the heart.

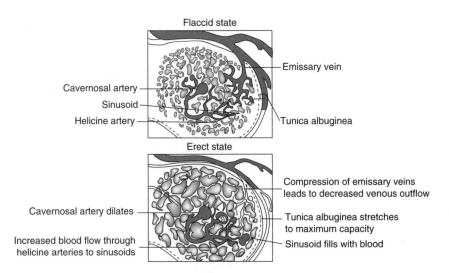

Figure 29   Mechanisms of normal erectile response.

nerves in his pelvis release chemicals that increase blood flow into the penis. The corpora cavernosa are similar to a sponge: just as a sponge absorbs liquids into its air spaces and distends when submerged, the corpora cavernosa have hollow spaces, or sinusoids, that distend with blood when sexual excitement causes increased blood flow to the penis. As the sinusoids fill with blood and distend, they compress the veins against the tunica albuginea. It is this compression of the veins that prevents blood from draining out of the penis, which promotes full rigidity and maintenance of the rigidity (Figure 29).

You might be surprised to learn that erections aren't simply something that happens in the penis. For an erection to occur, there must be proper functioning of many physical structures and systems: the brain, certain **nerves** in the **pelvis**, and the arteries and veins that supply the penis. When a man is aroused, the brain tells nerves in the pelvis to release neurotransmitters, which in turn stimulate the blood vessels in the penis to open up and the smooth muscle in the corpora cavernosa to relax to increase blood flow into the penis. After sexual performance is completed, the brain releases other chemicals that tell the arteries in the penis to constrict, thus decreasing blood flow to the penis and allowing the veins to drain the blood out of the penis. These chemicals that cause constriction of smooth muscle may also be released during times of stress and may adversely affect erectile function.

Now that you know that the erectile process is a neurovascular event, then it becomes clear that any disease process that affects the brain, the nerves in the pelvis,

Nerve

A cordlike structure composed of a collection of nerve fibers that conveys impulses between a part of the central nervous system and some other region of the body.

Pelvis

The part of the body that is framed by the hip bones.

the arteries to and within the penis, the veins in the penis, the tunica albuginea, or the erectile tissue within the corpora cavernosa may affect erectile function.

65. What is erectile dysfunction (ED) and how common is it?

The National Institutes of Health (NIH) definition of erectile dysfunction (ED), previously called impotence, is the consistent inability to achieve and/or maintain an erection satisfactory for the completion of sexual performance. The definition is subjective, meaning that the individual (and/or his partner) is the person who decides that his erections are not satisfactory. This is in comparison to an objective definition, in which an observer or a test makes the decision that the erection is not satisfactory. The definition is not an all-or-nothing one, meaning that different men may experience different degrees of ED. The most severe form of ED would be the complete absence of erections—no nocturnal (nighttime) erections, morning erections, or erections noted with stimulation; milder forms may be associated with inadequate degree or duration of rigidity.

The Massachusetts Male Aging Study was probably the first study that brought to light how common ED is. This study demonstrated that 52% of men between the ages of 40 years and 70 years have some degree of ED (**Figure 30**). Of those individuals, 10% noted complete ED, 25% noted moderate ED, and most noted mild ED.

In the United States, approximately 50 million men suffer from ED. The prevalence (number of cases of a

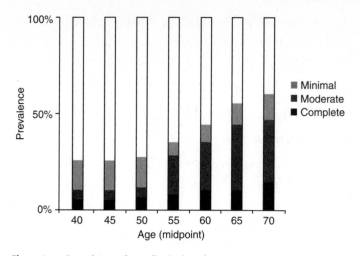

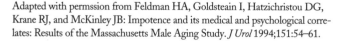

Figure 30   Prevalence of erectile dysfunction.

Adapted with permssion from Feldman HA, Goldsteain I, Hatzichristou DG, Krane RJ, and McKinley JB: Impotence and its medical and psychological corre-lates: Results of the Massachusetts Male Aging Study. *J Urol* 1994;151:54–61.

disease that are present at a given point in time) of ED is age dependent, with the rate of complete ED increasing from 5% among men 40 years old to 15% among those 70 years old. As our population continues to grow and age, we can only expect this number to increase. The worldwide prevalence of ED was 152 million in 1995 and is expected to increase to 322 million in 2025. Much of this increase will occur in the developing world and reflects the aging of the world's population.

The incidence (i.e., the number of new cases occurring during a specific period of time) of ED is higher in men with certain diseases, such as diabetes mellitus, hypertension, cardiovascular disease, spinal cord injury, and hypercholesterolemia (high cholesterol levels).

ED is a form of sexual dysfunction. The term sexual dysfunction applies to a variety of problems with sex, so the two terms are not really interchangeable (see Question 67). It is important that you determine early in your visit with your doctor whether your problem is ED and not another type of sexual dysfunction.

ED is not a disease in and of itself; rather, it is a manifestation of an underlying medical condition. It is important to evaluate men with ED to identify the underlying disease process(es) that is causing this problem because it may be a symptom (i.e., subjective evidence) of a condition that could cause the individual further harm. In addition, by treating the underlying disease processes, one may hopefully prevent further progression of the ED.

66. What causes ED?

Many medical conditions and medications (**Table 16**) can cause ED. Smoking, alcohol abuse, drug abuse, stress, and depression can also cause ED. Considering erectile function as a neurovascular event, we can divide the causes of ED into those that affect the brain and nerves (neurologic) and those that affect the arteries and veins (vascular).

Neurologic Conditions That Cause ED

A variety of neurologic conditions can cause ED. The most common of these are spinal cord injury, lumbar disk disease, stroke, Parkinson's disease, multiple sclerosis, Alzheimer's disease, and pituitary disease (pituitary adenoma). In addition, certain surgical procedures, such as radical prostatectomy for prostate cancer and surgery for rectal cancer, can injure the pelvic nerves. The incidence

Table 16   Medications That May Cause Erectile Dysfunction

Antidepressants and Other Psychiatric Medications	High Blood Pressure Medications and Diuretics	Anithistamines	Drugs to treat Parkinson's Disease	Chemotherapy and Hormonal Agents	Other Medications
Amitriptyline (Elavil)	Atenolol (Tenormin)	Cimetidine (Tagamet)	Benztropine (Cogentin)	Antiandrogens (Casodex, Flutamide, Nilutamide)	Aminocaproic acid (Amicar)
Amoxapine (Asendin)	Bethanidine	Dimenhydrinate (Dramamine)	Biperidin (Akineton)	Cyclophosphamide (Cytoxan)	Atropine
Buspirone (Buspar)	Bumetanide (Bumex)	Diphenhydramine (Benadryl)	Bromocriptine (Parlodel)	Ketoconazole	Clofibrate (Atromid-S)
Chlordiazepoxide (Librium)	Captopril (Capoten)	Hydroxyzine (Vis-taril)	Levodopa (Sinemet)	LHRH agonists (Lupron, Zoladex)	Cyclobenzaprine (Flexeril)
Chlorpromazine (Thorazine)	Chlorothiazide (Diuril)	Meclizine (Antivert)	Procyclidine (Kemadrin)	LHRH antagonist (Degarelix)	Cyproterone
Clomipramine (Anafril)	Chlorthalidone (Hygroton)	Nizatidine (Axid)	Trihexyphenidyl (Artane)		Digoxin (Lanoxin)
Clorazepate (Tranxene)	Clonidine (Catapres)	Promethazine (Phenergan)			Disopyramide (Norpace)
Desipramine (Norpramin)	Enalapril (Vasotec)	H2 blockers (Tagamet, Zantac, Pepcid)			Estrogen
Diazepam (Valium)	Furosemide (Lasix)				Finasteride (Propecia, Proscar, Avodart)

Erectile Dysfunction (ED)

Table 16   Medications That May Cause Erectile Dysfunction (Continued)

Antidepressants and Other Psychiatric Medications	High Blood Pressure Medications and Diuretics	Anithistamines	Drugs to treat Parkinson's Disease	Chemotherapy and Hormonal Agents	Other Medications
Doxepin (Sinequan)	Guanabenz (Wytensin)		Opiate analgesics		Furazolidone (Furoxone)
Fluoxetine (Prozac)	Guanethidine (Ismelin)		Codeine		Indomethacin (Indocin)
Fluphenazine (Prolixin)	Guanfacine (Tenex)		Fentanyl (Innovar)		Lipid lowering agents
Imipramine (Tofranil)	Haloperidol (Haldol)		Hydromorphone (Dilaudid)		Licorice
Isocarboxazid (Marplan)	Hydralazine (Apresoline)		Meperidine (Demerol)		Metoclopramide (Reglan)
Lorazepam (Ativan)	Hydrochlorothiazide (Esidrix)		Methadone		NSAIDS (Ibuprofen, etc)
Meprobamate (Equanil)	Labetalol (Normodyne)		Morphine		Orphenadrine (Norflex)
Mesoridazine (Serentil)	Methyldopa (Aldomet)		Oxycodone (Oxycontin, Percodan)		Prochlorperazine (Compazine)
Nortriptyline (Pamelor)	Metoprolol (Lopressor)				Pseudoephedrine (Sudafed)

(Continued)

173

Table 16 Medications That May Cause Erectile Dysfunction (*Continued*)

Antidepressants and Other Psychiatric Medications	High Blood Pressure Medications and Diuretics	Anithistamines	Drugs to treat Parkinson's Disease	Chemotherapy and Hormonal Agents	Other Medications
Oxazepam (Serax)	Minoxidil (Loniten)				
Phenelzine (Nardil)	Nifedipine (Adalat, Procardia)		Recreational Drugs		
Phenytoin (Dilantin)	Phenoxybenzamine (Dibenzyline)		Alcohol		
Sertraline (Zoloft)	Phentolamine (Regitine)		Amphetamines		
Thioridazine (Mellaril)	Prazosin (Minipress)		Barbiturates		
Thiothixene (Navane)	Propranolol (Inderal)		Cocaine		
Tranylcypromine (Parnate)	Reserpine (Serpasil)		Marijuana		
Trifluoperazine (Stelazine)	Spironolactone (Aldactone)		Heroin		
	Triamterene (Maxzide)		Nicotine		
	Verapamil (Calan)				

of ED after radical prostatectomy varies according to whether the patient experienced ED before surgery and whether a nerve-sparing procedure was performed. Reported rates of ED after bilateral nerve-sparing radical prostatectomy range from 18 to 82%. Other factors unrelated to disease or surgery can also cause ED. For example, long-distance bicycle riding on bicycles with small, hard seats has been implicated as a cause of ED, possibly by nerve or vascular compression.

Vascular Conditions That Cause ED

From a vascular standpoint, any disease process that can affect arteries may also affect the arteries that supply the penis. Men with coronary artery disease (sometimes manifested as angina, which is a pain in the chest, with a feeling of suffocation), cerebrovascular disease (which may have caused prior stroke or transient ischemic attack), peripheral vascular disease (decreased blood flow to the legs, often associated with aches/cramps in the legs when attempting to walk for a distance), high blood pressure, and high cholesterol levels are at increased risk for erectile troubles. Men who have experienced severe pelvic or perineal trauma, such as from a motor vehicle accident causing a pelvic fracture or direct injury to the penis, are at risk for ED.

Radiation therapy (administration of radiation to kill cancer cells) to the pelvis for colon cancer or prostate cancer can cause damage to the blood vessels supplying the penis. ED has been reported in 15 to 65% of men undergoing external-beam radiation therapy (high-energy radiation beams passed through the skin) for

For example, long–distance bicycle riding on bicycles with small, hard seats has been implicated as a cause of ED, possibly by nerve or vascular compression.

prostate cancer. The onset of ED after radiation therapy is usually not immediate; it typically occurs 2 or more years after the radiation therapy. Interstitial seed therapy for prostate cancer also affects erectile function in 25 to 60% of men who undergo it. As with external-beam radiation therapy, the effect on erectile function is usually seen a year or more after seed placement. Smoking causes vasospasm, or tightening up of the arteries, but it also may cause atherosclerosis, or hardening of the arteries. Venous leaks or abnormal veins may result from prior trauma and may be identified in Peyronie's disease, a benign condition affecting the penis in middle-aged men (see Questions 73 and 74).

Other Conditions That Cause ED

ED occurs to different degrees in different medical conditions. For example, erectile dysfunction occurs in about 27% of men with hypertension. The Massachusetts Male Aging Study found an association between low concentration of high-density lipoproteins (HDL—the good cholesterol) and ED, even though there was no correlation between ED and total cholesterol levels. (Cholesterol is a fatlike substance that is important to certain body functions but, when present in excessive amounts, contributes to unhealthy fatty deposits in the arteries, which may interfere with blood flow.) In men between the ages of 40 years and 55 years, the risk of moderate ED increased from 6.7 to 25% when the HDL level decreased from 90 to 30 mg/dL. This study also found a similar effect of the HDL level on erectile function in the older male population. Another study did find a relationship between the total cholesterol and erectile function; according to this study, the risk of ED increased as total cholesterol level increased.

This study also found a negative correlation between HDL level and risk of ED—meaning that the higher the HDL level, the lower the risk of ED. This increased risk of ED with low HDL levels and elevated cholesterol levels is not surprising, because these are the factors that increase one's risk of cardiovascular disease.

Another condition in which ED commonly occurs is diabetes mellitus. An estimated 15.7 million people in the United States have diabetes, including 7.5 million men. Type 2 diabetes, also called noninsulin-dependent diabetes mellitus, accounts for 90–95% of the patients with diabetes mellitus; type 1 diabetes, or insulin-dependent diabetes mellitus, accounts for 5–10%. The prevalence of ED in diabetes ranges from 35 to 75%. In men with treated diabetes mellitus in the Massachusetts Male Aging Study, the age-adjusted prevalence of complete ED (no erections at any time) was 28%, which was about three times higher than the prevalence of complete ED in the entire sample of men in the Massachusetts Male Aging Study.

ED occurs in a large number (82%) of men on hemodialysis for renal (kidney) failure. Men on hemodialysis are more likely to experience ED if they are older, if they have diabetes mellitus, and if they do not use angiotensin-converting enzyme (ACE) inhibitors. The cause of the ED is probably multifactorial; it may be partly related to the medical condition that caused the renal failure (e.g., diabetes mellitus), but it also may be related to hormonal changes that occur with dialysis. Dialysis patients have lower testosterone levels and may have high prolactin levels. In addition, dialysis lowers zinc levels and may cause overactivity of the parathyroid gland (hyperparathyroidism).

Smoking may be an independent risk factor for ED, particularly erectile dysfunction caused by vascular disease, and it may also contribute to other causes of ED. In the Massachusetts Male Aging Study, neither the number of cigarettes smoked nor the duration of time smoking had an effect on the incidence of ED. However, the study did show a significant relationship between smoking and erectile dysfunction for certain categories of men. In men who were being treated for heart disease, complete ED was 56% for current smokers, compared with 21% for nonsmokers, after correction for differences in age. Similar results were noted for men with high blood pressure (20% incidence of erectile dysfunction in current smokers versus 8.5% in nonsmokers), those with arthritis (20% in current smokers versus 9.4% in nonsmokers), those taking heart medications (41% in current smokers versus 14% in nonsmokers), and those taking medications for high blood pressure (21% for current smokers versus 7.5% in nonsmokers).

Where alcohol use is concerned, as the saying goes, "Too much of a good thing is bad." Alcohol is thought of as a relaxant, and its use will take away one's inhibitions. Yet alcohol abuse—regular drinking to excess—can cause ED; occasional use does not. Liver failure as a result of alcohol abuse may also affect erectile function.

Purely psychogenic (originating from the mind or psyche) ED probably accounts for only 10% of the patients with ED. Depression, anxiety, and stress may have an adverse effect on erectile function, and many of the medications used to treat these problems can cause ED and other forms of sexual dysfunction. However, in most situations, once erectile dysfunction occurs the man develops psychogenic components related to the anxieties that ED causes. Psychogenic causes of ED include:

- Performance anxiety
- Depression
- Marital problems
- Dysfunctional attitude toward sex
- Sexual phobia
- Religious beliefs/inhibitions
- Prior traumatic sexual experience

A variety of other medical conditions have been associated with ED, including endocrine abnormalities, such as hyperthyroidism (overactive thyroid gland), hypothyroidism (underactive thyroid gland), hypogonadism (when the testes don't produce enough testosterone), and pituitary dysfunction (sometimes manifested by hyperprolactinemia, or excess prolactin production).

Medications that Cause ED

Hypertension (high blood pressure) may be a risk factor for ED, and several blood pressure medications (antihypertensives) have been described as causing ED. Most notably beta-blockers, such as metoprolol, atenolol, and labetolol, and thiazide diuretics, such as hydrochlorothiazide. The only thiazide diuretic that has not been associated with ED is indapamide.

Clonidine (Catapres), another blood pressure medication, is also associated with an increased incidence of ED.

The incidence of ED in patients taking antidepressants has been reported to be as high as 35%. Tricyclic antidepressants, such as imipramine (Tofranil), amitriptyline (Elavil), protriptyline (Concordin), and clomipramine (Anafranil), have been reported to cause ED. It appears that they affect ejaculatory function more than erectile function. Selective serotonin reuptake inhibitors (SSRIs) were initially thought to have less of an effect on erectile function; however, studies suggest that 50% of men who are taking SSRIs may experience ED. There have been reports of ED being associated with fluvoxamine (Luvox), fluoxetine (Prozac), sertraline (Zoloft), and paroxetine (Paxil). In rare cases, ED has improved with SSRI use. Antipsychotics such as thioridazine (Mellaril), fluphenazine (Prolixin), and thiothixene (Navane) have also been associated with ED, with up to 44% men taking thioridazine reporting ED. Benzodiazepines, used to treat such conditions as posttraumatic stress disorder, may also cause ED. Clonazepam (Klonopin) use has been associated with a 43% incidence of ED, whereas the other benzodiazepines and the tranquilizers diazepam (Valium), lorazepam (Ativan), and alprazolam (Xanax) have not been associated with ED.

Cimetidine (Tagamet), a histamine$_2$-antagonist used for gastrointestinal irritation, has been reported to cause ED in 40% of men. It is known to prevent testosterone from functioning and may also increase prolactin levels, which can lower testosterone levels, decrease libido, and affect erectile function. The other histamine$_2$-antagonists, ranitidine (Zantac) and famotidine (Pepcid), do not have the same effect on testosterone and are not as frequently associated with ED.

Medications used to lower one's cholesterol (lipid) level such as clofibrate (Atromid-S), gemfibrozil (Lopid), pravastatin (Pravachol) and lovastatin (Mevacor) may also affect erectile function. Digoxin, a cardiac medication, has also been associated with ED, as have the seizure medications phenytoin (Dilantin), carbamazepine (Tegretol), primidone (Mysoline), and phenobarbitol (10 to 20% incidence).

Hormone therapies for prostate cancer, such as leuprolide (Lupron) and goserelin (Zoladex), orchiectomy, and estrogen, have a negative effect on erectile function. Recreational drugs, including alcohol, cocaine, marijuana, and heroin, may also have a negative effect on erectile function. Up to 50 to 80% of alcoholics experience ED; the ED may resolve with prolonged abstinence, but in some men it may persist. Marijuana decreases testosterone levels, and long-term marijuana use may affect erectile function. Opiate addiction is commonly associated with loss of libido (interest in sex) and ED. With abstinence from opiates, the ED improves. Anabolic steroids, used by body builders and athletes to increase their muscle mass, cause testicular atrophy and decrease testosterone production, which may decrease sperm production, decrease libido, and cause ED. If the anabolic steroids are discontinued, it may take 4 months for the testicles to start producing enough testosterone to restore erectile function to normal. The medication ketoconazole, if taken in large quantities, may also affect testosterone production and affect erectile function.

67. Is ED a normal process of aging? Is ED preventable? Is it curable?

Older men often note that it takes longer to achieve an erection. In fact, men older than 50 years can take 2 to 3 times longer to develop an erection than younger men. The erection may not be as rigid as in younger years, and arousal alone may not lead to full rigidity without tactile (touch) stimulation. It may also take longer to climax. Ejaculation (the release of semen through the penis during orgasm) may not occur, or it may occur with less force. The recovery period after ejaculation increases with age, and many men older than 55 years are not able to have another erection for 12 to 24 hours after ejaculating. These normal changes related to aging should not be confused with sexual dysfunction or ED; failure to understand these normal changes and to adapt to them may cause stress and anxiety and may complicate erectile function. In ED, the erections are either inadequate for penetration or do not last long enough for completion of sexual performance. In short, the incidence of ED does increase with age, but it is not an expected process of aging.

Age-related changes in sexual function do occur and include a decrease in the amount of smooth muscle in the penis, which may affect erectile function. The sensitivity of the penis can also decrease with age, so that more stimulation is required for an erection. In men older than 60 years, levels of free testosterone in the bloodstream (the active form of testosterone) often decline. Chronic illnesses, which are more common in the elderly, also may decrease testosterone levels, which could affect the vascular response to sexual arousal and libido.

Other factors that aren't necessarily restricted to older men can compound age-related changes; for example, morbid obesity and excessive alcohol consumption over a long period of time decrease testosterone levels.

Is ED preventable?

Many medical conditions that can cause ED are inherited, so, at this point in time, we cannot prevent them. However, conditions such as hypertension, high cholesterol, and diabetes mellitus can be improved by lifestyle changes, such as exercise and proper diet. If you have diabetes mellitus, tight control of your blood sugar level may not totally prevent the occurrence of ED, but it may prevent the ED from progressing. Avoiding excessive alcohol intake and smoking may also help to decrease your risk of ED. Similarly, if you are a long-distance bicycle rider and experience genital numbness when you finish a bike ride, you may want to start using a bicycle seat designed to put less pressure on the perineum.

Is ED curable?

In most cases, ED is not curable—but usually it is treatable. Steps can be taken to help a man have erections—that's what is meant by treatment—but these steps cannot reverse the underlying causes of the dysfunction, which is what is meant by curing a problem. However, in select instances, ED is curable. For example, in young, otherwise healthy men who suffer an acute injury to one of the penile arteries that leads to narrowing or blockage of the artery, a surgical procedure may be performed to reestablish blood flow to the penis. Penile arterial bypass surgery, similar to arterial bypass surgery performed for blocked blood vessels to the heart or the legs, can be performed for damage to penile arteries. Candidates for penile arterial bypass surgery must have only an arterial cause of their ED. There must be no evidence of any other causes of their ED, such as venous leak, neurologic problems, or hormonal abnormalities. In addition, they should not have any underlying disease processes that would adversely affect the bypass, such as elevated cholesterol, diabetes, and high blood pressure, and they may not smoke.

Previously potent men who undergo a nerve-sparing radical prostatectomy and experience postoperative erectile dysfunction may experience a return of their erectile function during the first 2 years after their surgery. Treating the ED early and increasing the penile blood flow may improve erectile function. Finally, men with a psychogenic cause may note resolution of their ED with appropriate treatment of their psychological problems.

Where surgery and psychotherapy aren't able to resolve the problem, other treatment methods, such as medical therapy (oral, intraurethral, and intracavernous) and mechanical devices (the vacuum device or a prosthesis, i.e., a device used to replace the lost normal function of a structure or organ) can help most men achieve a satisfactory erection when desired (Question 75).

68. What is sexual dysfunction?

The term "sexual dysfunction" broadly encompasses trouble with any component of the sexual response cycle. The sexual response cycle in men consists of sexual desire/interest (libido), sexual arousal (erection), orgasm (including emission [involuntary discharge of semen from the ejaculatory duct into the urethra] and ejaculation), and detumescence (return of the penis to the flaccid, nonerect state). An abnormality in one component of the sexual response cycle may not affect the remainder of the components of the cycle. For example, one may still be able to climax and ejaculate without achieving a rigid erection. Common sexual dysfunctions include problems with libido, ejaculation, and orgasm.

Libido

Lack of interest in sex is often called decreased libido or decreased desire. Libido is governed by psychogenic factors and involves all five senses (sight, smell, taste, touch, and hearing) as well as hormonal factors. Low libido, or hypoactive sexual desire, occurs in about 15% of men and in about 20% of the general population, both men and women. Depression and anxiety may adversely affect one's libido, and depression is the leading cause of hypoactive sexual desire. Other causes of hypoactive desire include relationship factors: lack of trust, intimacy conflicts, and lack of physical attraction to one's partner. The hormone testosterone is the main hormone responsible for libido in men. Testosterone levels have an effect on libido and on sexual thoughts and fantasies.

Sexual Arousal (Erection)

Sexual arousal requires input from nerves and arteries. To achieve an adequate erection, there must be at least six times as much blood flow into the corpora cavernosa. Changes in nerves, arteries, and veins may lead to trouble with erections. The Massachusetts male aging study demonstrated that approximately 52% of males have some degree of erectile dysfunction between the ages of 40 and 70.

Ejaculation

Ejaculatory dysfunction includes premature ejaculation, retrograde ejaculation, delayed ejaculation, and anejaculation. Premature ejaculation means that ejaculation occurs too quickly and may occur with light stimulation before, on, or shortly after penetration, or simply before one wishes for it to occur. Retrograde ejaculation is a condition in which the ejaculate passes backward into the bladder; this condition may be associated with decreased ejaculate volume or no ejaculate. Delayed ejaculation is a condition in which it takes too long to ejaculate; it is frequently associated with the use of the newer antidepressants, the SSRIs. Anejaculation is a condition in which no ejaculation occurs at all.

Orgasm

Orgasm is another term used for sexual climax, or the culmination of sexual excitement. Orgasmic dysfunction refers to alterations in orgasmic function or the inability to achieve an orgasm, to climax. Anorgasmia (complete absence of orgasm) occurs in 17% of married men and affects younger men more commonly. Psychological causes of anorgasmia include fear of pregnancy or AIDS, anxiety disorders, and repressive cultural, parental, or religious attitudes toward sexuality.

Anorgasmia (complete absence of orgasm) occurs in 17% of married men and affects younger men more commonly.

69. How does one diagnose and evaluate ED?

The diagnosis (identification of the cause or presence of a medical problem or disease) and evaluation of ED require a thorough history, complete physical examination, and possibly some laboratory testing. At first, your doctor will want to establish that the problem truly is ED and not some other form of sexual dysfunction (see Question 68). Your doctor may start the visit out by first paraphrasing the definition of ED—the consistent inability to achieve and/or maintain an erection satisfactory for the completion of sexual performance—to make sure that you are both discussing the same problem. Your doctor will also need a history, which will involve asking a number of questions about your medical, social, and sexual background. Some of these questions might be uncomfortable or embarrassing, but you should answer them as honestly as possible because this is probably the most important part of the diagnostic process, allowing the physician to identify common risk factors for both organic (having a physical origin) and psychogenic (originating from the mind or psyche) erectile dysfunction.

What questions might the doctor ask me during my initial visit?

Questions such as the following will help evaluate the cause and the magnitude of the erectile dysfunction:

- How long have you been experiencing ED?
- Was the onset abrupt or a slow, progressive deterioration in function?
- Can you identify a precipitating event?
- Is the problem constant or intermittent?
- Does it occur with only one partner or with all partners if there are multiple partners?
- Do you achieve any erection with stimulation, and do you notice nocturnal or evening erections?
- Do you get an erection that is rigid enough for penetration?
- Does your erection last long enough for completion of sexual performance?
- Is there any penile pain or curvature associated with erections?
- What medical conditions do you have?
- Have you had any prior surgery?
- Do you take any medications?
- Do you smoke?
- Do you drink alcohol, and if so, how much?
- Do you use any recreational drugs?
- Do you feel stressed or depressed?
- Is the ED causing you to feel stressed or depressed?
- Is your partner interested in restoring your sexual relationship?

Often, your physician may ask you to complete a questionnaire: the International Index of Erectile Function, or IIEF (see Appendix A), an abbreviated question-naire called the Brief Sexual Function Inventory (BSFI), or the Sexual Health Inventory for Men (SHIM), an abbreviated IIEF that contains five questions (see Appendix A). These questionnaires are helpful in assessing your problem and also may help assess your response to therapies.

What is the doctor looking for during the physical examination?

The physical examination looks for clinical signs of several disorders including hypertension, cardiovascular disease, renal or liver disease, peripheral vascular disease, thyroid problems, and neurologic problems that may be causing your ED. It is a head-to-toe examination in which your doctor will look at:

- Your heart rate and blood pressure to determine whether there might be a vascular problem.
- Your head and neck to rule out yellow sclera (liver failure) and to check for thyroid enlargement and swollen lymph nodes.
- Your chest to see how well your lungs and heart are working and to look for gynecomastia (tender or enlarged breasts in males, which can be a sign of a pituitary problem).
- Your abdomen, which will be examined by palpation (feeling with the hand or fingers, by applying light pressure), to rule out enlarged liver or kidneys, abdominal masses, or tenderness.
- Your genitalia (external sexual organs) to make sure that there are no plaques or abnormalities of the penis; the doctor will also check the testes to make sure that both are present, of normal size, and have no tumors and will check secondary sex characteristics, such as pubic hair.

- Your femoral pulse, located in your thigh, and pulses in your feet to rule out peripheral vascular disease.
- Your penile sensation, reflexes, and rectal tone. This may be uncomfortable: the doctor will check the bulbocavernosus reflex by inserting a finger in your rectum, squeezing the tip of penis, and noting a contraction of the anus at time of squeezing penis.

Why is my doctor checking my testosterone level?

There are several reasons why your doctor will check a testosterone level during your initial evaluation. First, rare benign pituitary tumors can lower testosterone production and cause decreased libido and ED. These tumors are treatable, and the sexual side effects are potentially reversible. Second, if you have decreased libido, the doctor is attempting to determine whether supplemental testosterone can improve poor libido. There is no other way of assessing your testosterone level besides the blood test because neither libido nor testis size is a good gauge of testosterone levels. Clearly, if you have a decrease in your libido and your testosterone level is low, then supplemental testosterone will enhance your libido. However, in some patients with ED, who fail oral therapy and have a low normal serum testosterone, the use of supplemental testosterone may enhance the response to oral therapy, despite having normal libido.

What happens after the history, physical examination, and laboratory tests have been carried out?

In most cases, once possible causes have been identified and evaluated, your doctor may discuss lifestyle changes and possible therapies with you. This goal-oriented approach centers around the doctor and patient discussing possible origins of the problem and then making a decision about therapy (**Figure 31**). In select cases, when

Evaluation and Treatment of Men with Erectile Dysfunction

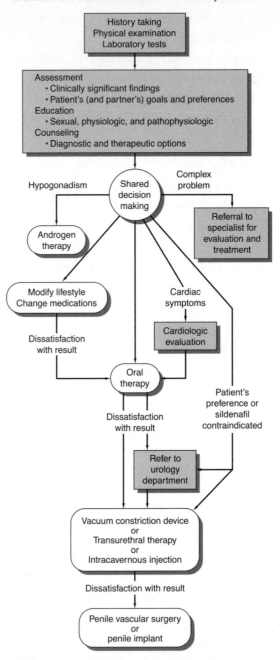

Figure 31   Approach to the evaluation and treatment of erectile dysfunction.

Adapted with permission from *N Engl J Med* 2000;342:1807. Copyright © 2000, The Massachusetts Medical Society.

the patient wants to know more about the cause of the ED—is it really an artery problem or a vein problem?—then further investigation is required. Young men with no identifiable medical conditions or risk factors should undergo further evaluation because these individuals are the best candidates for penile vascular surgery.

If there appears to be a significant psychological component to the ED then it may be appropriate to seek consultation with a psychiatrist, psychologist, or sex therapist. Although organic problems account for 80 to 90% of the cases of ED, realistically, in many men there is some psychological overlay. Treating the ED may resolve psychological problems related to ED, but if there are significant psychological stressors, then psychological counseling at the same time as medical therapy may be more beneficial than medical therapy alone.

It is important to identify possible causes of your ED so that you and your doctor can find the best method of treating it. The success rates of many therapies have been subdivided based on the causes and the degree of ED. Knowing where your problem comes from will allow you to determine the likelihood of success of a given therapy and to avoid falsely elevated expectations.

It is often very helpful if your partner can participate in the evaluation and treatment process. Realistically, an intervention is unlikely to succeed if your partner is not interested in resuming sexual relations. For example, if your partner is a postmenopausal woman, she might suffer from atrophic vaginitis, which stems from lower estrogen levels that cause the vaginal mucosa to become thin, dry, and prone to irritation. If this is the case, she may find intercourse uncomfortable—and you may not

It is often very helpful if your partner can participate in the evaluation and treatment process.

have a supportive partner to help you through the therapy for your ED. This might be an opportunity to address both problems; discomfort from atrophic vaginitis can be improved by using lubricants during intercourse. In addition, the use of topical estrogen cream helps restore the vaginal mucosa in women for whom such agents are appropriate, so your partner may want to discuss with her primary care provider or gynecologist the risks and benefits of topical estrogen therapy for atrophic vaginitis.

What laboratory tests are performed?

The laboratory evaluation of ED is limited in most cases. If you are treated by a primary care provider on a regular basis, such information as a fasting blood sugar test, kidney function tests, liver function tests, and lipid profile are often available. If you have experienced unexplainable weight gain or loss and/or other signs or symptoms of abnormal thyroid function, then thyroid function tests may be performed. All men with ED should have a serum testosterone level checked. Because the testosterone level varies throughout the day and tends to be highest in the morning, it is best to have the testosterone level checked in the morning. In some men, such as obese men and those with liver disease, the total testosterone level may be low, but the free testosterone level (the active form of testosterone) is normal. If the testosterone level is low, then a prolactin level should be checked to rule out a pituitary adenoma (a benign brain tumor).

Do I need any specialized tests?

In most cases, the history, physical examination, and blood testing allow the physician to identify possible causes of your ED, but in some cases, a more advanced evaluation may be required. In men who seem to have a psychogenic basis for their problem, the doctor might order nocturnal penile tumescence (NPT) studies to confirm this theory. (Tumescence is the state of being swollen, in this case referring to having an erection.) This test involves wearing a specialized device around the penis at night on several occasions when sleeping. The device records whether you have erections during your sleep, which is both normal and common; if you do, it would suggest that the ED could be psychogenic in origin, which can help determine the correct treatment strategy. However, NPT studies have limitations, and it has been suggested that sleep-related erections may not be the same as sexually induced erections.

If your doctor wishes to evaluate your penile vasculature and obtain a preliminary assessment of the arterial and venous function therein, the best initial test is **Doppler ultrasonography** in conjunction with injection therapy. In ultrasound studies, internal organs are visualized by measurement of reflected sound waves. In this particular study, you are injected with a chemical that causes smooth muscle relaxation and increases penile blood flow, usually 10 μg of alprostadil (Caverject, Edex), but other agents, such as trimix/triple P (prostaglandin E_1, papaverine, and phentolamine), may be used. After injection, sequential blood flow studies are performed. The rate at which blood is flowing through the cavernosal artery on each side of the penis (the peak systolic velocity) can be determined. A peak systolic velocity over 25 to 30 mL/sec is considered normal. The Doppler ultrasound also allows the diameter of the cavernosal arteries to be measured. In addition, the function of the penile veins can be assessed by measuring the end-diastolic velocity (venous resistance). The Doppler ultrasound study may be affected by patient anxiety and may require stimulation to achieve the maximum

Doppler ultrasonography

Use of a Doppler probe during ultrasound to look at flow through vessels.

response. As with injection therapy, there is a small risk of priapism and penile pain related to the injection or to the medication used. If the Doppler ultrasound study demonstrates an abnormality of the arteries or veins and the patient wishes to be evaluated for possible surgical correction, then further studies would be required. **Arteriography**, or **cavernosography** are performed to better assess possible arterial or venous abnormalities. These more invasive tests are not required in all individuals and should be performed in select institutions where penile artery bypass surgery or venous ligation surgery is performed.

What are nocturnal penile tumescence (NPT) studies?

Formal nocturnal penile tumescence (NPT) testing requires spending two to three consecutive nights in the sleep laboratory. Men undergoing NPT tests must abstain from alcohol, caffeine, and medications that may affect sleep or erections for 8 hours before the test. Because sleep erections occur primarily during rapid eye movement (REM) sleep, one must assess the quality of REM sleep, which is done through the use of an electroencephalographic (EEG) test, an electro-oculographic test, and a submental electromyographic test. To assess penile tumescence, two mercury-in-rubber strain gauges (expandable rubber loops) are placed on the penis, one at the base and the other just behind the glans penis. When the loop circumferences increase, the mercury column is thinned, this increases the electrical resistance through the mercury. Each time there is an increase in the electrical resistance, it is recorded on a tracing. The high point of the deflection on the tracing corresponds to the change in penile circumference. The study also allows one to detect discrepancies between the changes in both loops, meaning that if one loop expands

Arteriography

A test for identifying and locating arterial disease in the penis, using injection of contrast into the arteries supplying the penis to look for areas of "blockage."

Cavernosography

A technique used to visualize areas of venous leak. It involves the injection of a cavernous smooth-muscle dilator (e.g., prostaglandin E_1 or trimix), followed by placement of a butterfly needle into the corpora, instillation of a contrast agent into the corpora, and X-ray photographs to visualize the sites of venous leak.

substantially more than the other, the test can detect this. One of the biggest drawbacks of NPTs is that they are measuring nocturnal erections, not erections related to sexual arousal, and each may occur via different mechanisms. Secondly, there can be false-positive NPT results; these more commonly occur in patients with neurogenic ED and pelvic steal syndrome, and false-negative NPT results occur in patients with depression, alcohol use, medication ingestion, and **sleep apnea**. In addition, the measurements of penile rigidity with NPT studies may be insufficient to differentiate between organic and psychogenic erectile dysfunction. Formal nocturnal penile tumescence testing is also laborious and expensive.

Sleep apnea

A condition in which a person stops breathing for a short period of time during sleep (anywhere from a few seconds to a minute or two), causing him to wake repeatedly and get insufficient sleep.

What is the RigiScan?

The RigiScan (Timm Medical Technologies, Eden Prairie, MN) was developed as a portable home device to evaluate the quality and the quantity of nocturnal penile erections. It is used to provide continuous measurements of penile rigidity and tumescence, and it represents an improvement over previous techniques of assessing nocturnal penile tumescence. The RigiScan consists of a portable battery-powered unit that is strapped around the thigh and has two loops that are connected to a direct-current torque motor. One loop is placed around the base of the penis and the other is placed just below the corona (the area of the penis just before the glans penis). To measure tumescence every 30 seconds, the loops tighten and the penile circumference (loop length) is recorded. Fifteen seconds later, a second measurement is taken without active tightening of the loops. If tumescence (measured by the length of the loop) increases by 10 mm or more from the initial measurements, rigidity measurements are taken. Rigidity is measured every 30 seconds by a slight tightening of the loops. Rigidity is expressed as a percentage, with 100% equaling the rigidity of a noncompressible rubber shaft. Rigidity measurements are discontinued when tumescence decreases to within 10 mm of baseline. The RigiScan can record three uninterrupted 10-hour sessions. The information stored in the device can then be downloaded into a microprocessor, and the nocturnal penile tumescence and rigidity information can be analyzed, displayed, and printed. The RigiScan measures only radial rigidity, that is, rigidity across the width or circumference; it does not measure axial rigidity, or rigidity across the length of the penis. Axial rigidity is the most important measurement in predicting vaginal penetration because it is used to assess the ability of the penis to stay straight despite pressure against the tip.

Axial rigidity is the most important measurement in predicting vaginal penetration because it is used to assess the ability of the penis to stay straight despite pressure against the tip.

In most patients, the RigiScan device can distinguish functional from inadequate erections and is helpful in distinguishing psychogenic from organic ED.

70. What happens if my sex drive (libido) is low? What causes it, can it be treated?

Sex hormones

Substances (estrogens and androgens) responsible for secondary sex characteristics (e.g., hair growth and voice change in males).

Your interest in sex is governed by **sex hormones**, primarily testosterone, and by psychosocial factors. Low testosterone levels are associated with decreased libido. Stress, depression, or anxiety may also affect your libido. In men with erectile dysfunction, interest in sex may be diminished as a result of their inability to achieve an adequate erection.

Any man with decreased libido should have his serum testosterone level checked. Normally, there is a feedback loop between the brain and the **testes**. The brain, through the release of luteinizing hormone (LH), tells the testicles to produce testosterone. The production of testosterone by the testicles acts on the brain to decrease the release of LH. If the testicles don't produce enough testosterone, the brain releases more LH in an attempt to stimulate the testicles to produce more testosterone. If the brain does not release enough LH, the testicles won't produce enough testosterone. This problem may occur in men with brain tumors or congenital abnormalities.

Another problem that can affect testosterone production is overactivity of the pituitary gland. The pituitary gland is a gland in the brain that is comprised of an anterior lobe and a posterior lobe. The anterior lobe produces such hormones as luteinizing hormone and prolactin. Overactivity of the pituitary gland can be caused by a pituitary adenoma (benign [noncancerous] tumor of the pituitary gland). This abnormality can lead to an elevated prolactin level, which in turn suppresses testosterone production.

Abnormalities of the testicles themselves that lead to impaired function of the testes may cause the testosterone levels to be low. Such abnormalities may include a history of testicular torsion, a history of undescended testes, prior testicular infections, and other congenital anomalies that affect the testes. Removal of both testes (bilateral orchiectomy) for prostate cancer or (rarely) bilateral testicular cancers causes a significant drop in testosterone level and decreases libido. Men with a single testis usually have adequate testosterone production, provided that the remaining testis is normal.

Testis

One of two male reproductive organs that are located within the scrotum and produce testosterone and sperm.

Erectile Dysfunction (ED)

Testosterone levels do decrease as one ages, but this does not usually cause problems with libido.

If you have decreased libido and your testosterone level is low then you may benefit from testosterone replacement therapy (see Question 76). Men with prostate cancer on LHRH agonist hormonal therapy will have a low testosterone level and may suffer from associated low libido. In these men, testosterone replacement therapy is contraindicated, and there would need to be a conscious effort to think about sex. Similarly, individuals who are stressed or depressed may experience low libido, and if their testosterone level is normal, administration of testosterone replacement therapy would not be beneficial.

71. Are there different types of problems with ejaculation? What causes them and how are they treated?

There are three different types of ejaculatory problems that can occur: premature ejaculation, retrograde ejaculation, and anejaculation.

What is premature ejaculation and what causes it?

Premature ejaculation is ejaculation that occurs sooner than desired, either before or shortly after penetration, that causes distress to one or both partners. This condition tends to occur more frequently in younger men. Premature ejaculation is the most common form of sexual dysfunction, occurring in 21% of men ages 18 to 59 years in the United States. The condition may be lifelong (primary) or acquired (secondary). Despite its prevalence, men rarely seek help. Some men with ED may develop secondary premature ejaculation, possibly caused by either the need for intense stimulation to attain and maintain an erection or because of anxiety associated with difficulty in attaining and maintaining an erection. In these patients, treating the erectile dysfunction may lead to resolution of the premature ejaculation.

It appears that men with premature ejaculation may have an increased sensitivity and excitability of the glans penis and the dorsal nerve, which supplies sensation to the penis.

What is retrograde ejaculation and what causes it?

Retrograde ejaculation occurs when the ejaculate flows backward into the bladder instead of forward and out the tip of the penis. There are three potential causes of retrograde ejaculation:

1. Anatomic—that which occurs following surgery on the bladder neck or from a congenital process. Retrograde ejaculation is very common in men who have underdone a transurethral prostatectomy (**TURP**). A TURP is usually performed to treat benign enlargement of the prostate.

2. Neurologic—resulting from disorders that interfere with the ability of the bladder neck to close during emission such as diabetes mellitus or retroperitoneal surgery.

3. Pharmacologic—caused by paralysis of the bladder neck by certain medications. Such medications include the blood pressure medications phenoxybenzamine (Dibenzyline), phentolamine, prazosin (Minipress), and the antipsychotic medications thioridazine (Mellaril), chlorpromazine (Thorazine), triflupromazine (Vespein), and mesoridazine (Serentil). Tamsulosin (Flomax) was thought to cause

TURP

A surgical technique performed under anesthesia using a specialized instrument similar to the cystoscope that allows the surgeon to remove the prostatic tissue that is bulging into the urethra and blocking the flow of urine through the urethra. After a TURP, the outer rim of the prostate remains.

retrograde ejaculation but it appears to cause anejaculation.

Retrograde ejaculation does not cause any harm—one
simply urinates out the ejaculate.

What is anejaculation and what causes it?

Anejaculation is the condition in which there is no flow
of ejaculate in either direction. This condition occurs
in some men with spinal cord injuries and in some
men with cancer of the testis who have undergone surgery to remove affected lymph nodes, a procedure
called retroperitoneal lymph node dissection. Anejaculation may also occur if the outflow of the ejaculate is
blocked; this may be caused by a small stone in the
ejaculatory duct (the structure through which the ejaculate passes into the urethra), or by prior infection and
scarring of the male reproductive tract from sexually
transmitted diseases, such as gonorrhea, and other diseases that affect the genitourinary tract, including
tuberculosis. In such cases, the ejaculatory duct may be
opened surgically. Anejaculation occurs after a radical
prostatectomy because the seminal vesicles and prostate
gland are removed and the vas deferens is tied off.
Congenital disorders such as imperforate anus and their
treatment may also cause anejaculation. Tamsulosin is
thought to cause reversible anejaculation.

How are the different types of ejaculatory dysfunction
treated?

There are two main types of treatment available for the
management of premature ejaculation, behavioral therapy
and medical therapy (see **Table 17**). Behavioral therapy
starts with education regarding what premature ejaculation is and the possible causes as well as teaching the

Table 17 Pharmacologic Therapies Used to Treat Premature Ejaculation

Type	Oral Therapy	Trade Name	Recommended Dose	Side Effects
Nonselective (SRI)	Clomipramine	Anafranil	25 mg to 50 mg/day or 25 mg 4–24 hrs pre-intercourse	Dry mouth, drowsiness, decreased libido, potential drug-drug interactions, rarely mania and withdrawal sx
Selective (SSRIs)	Fluoxetine	Prozac	5 mg to 20 mg/day or 20 mg 3–4 hrs pre-intercourse	As above
	Paroxetine	Paxil	10 mg, 20 mg, or 40 mg/day or 20 mg 2–4 hrs pre-intercourse	As above
	Sertraline	Zoloft	25 mg– 200 mg/day or 50 mg 4–8 hrs pre-intercourse	As above
Topical therapy	Lidocaine/prilocaine cream	EMLA	lidocaine 2.5%/ prilocaine 2.5% 20 to 30 min pre-intercourse	Numbness, partner irritation or numbness, prolonged application may lead to loss of erection

male strategies to manage the premature ejaculation. The squeeze technique is the most common technique used to treat premature ejaculation. The male is instructed to interrupt sexual relations when he feels that he is about to experience premature orgasm and ejaculation. He or his partner then squeezes the shaft of the penis between a thumb and two fingers, applying light pressure for about 20 seconds, then letting go and resuming sexual relations. Behavioral therapy is successful in 60 to 90% of men with premature ejaculation, however, it requires the cooperation of both partners.

Although pharmacologic therapy is used in men with premature ejaculation, none of the medications currently used in the management of premature ejaculation have been approved by the FDA for this specific indication. Premature ejaculation can be treated effectively with serotonin reuptake inhibitors (SRIs) or topical anesthetics (Table 17). A variety of SRIs including fluoxetine, paroxetene, sertaline, and the tricyclic antidepressant, clomipramine have been used. SRIs have provided significant benefit over placebo in clinical trials.

PSD502 is a topical spray comprised of lidocaine 7.5 mg and prilocaine 3.5 mg that is under investigation for the treatment of premature ejaculation. Preliminary studies have demonstrated that it is superior to placebo.

The treatment options for retrograde ejaculation vary with the cause.

The treatment options for retrograde ejaculation vary with the cause. If the retrograde ejaculation is related to an anatomic abnormality, it is rarely treatable. If the retrograde ejaculation is the result of medications, it may resolve with discontinuation of the medication. It is important to check with your medical doctor prior to discontinuing any of your medications to ensure that it is safe to do so. Lastly, if the retrograde ejaculation is related to a neurologic problem, it may respond to pharmacologic therapy. Medications that have been used in the treatment of retrograde ejaculation are alpha-sympathomimetics, medications that stimulate the bladder neck to close. These medications include pseudoephedrine, ephedrine, phenylephrine, chlorpheniramine, bromphenramine, or imipramine. These medications may increase your blood pressure and your heart rate. Thus if you have any history of hypertension or heart disease it is important to check with your medical doctor before trying any of these medications.

With anejaculation, treatment is focused only on those men who wish to father a child. Electroejaculation (EEJ), the low-current stimulation of the ejaculatory organs via a rectal probe, can lead to emission in men with anejaculation. This form of treatment requires anesthesia in nonspinal cord injury males. Penile vibratory stimulation (PVS) may also be effective in spinal cord injury males.

72. What is anorgasmia and how is it treated?

Anorgasmia, the inability to achieve an orgasm, may be congenital or acquired. It is estimated that about 90% of anorgasmia problems are related to psychological issues. Surveys point to performance anxiety as a common psychological problem. There is a relationship between anorgasmia and childhood or adult sexual abuse or rape. Marital strife, boredom with a relationship, coupled with a monotonous sex life are other contributing factors. Some drugs, such as alcohol and the selective serotonin reuptake inhibitors may impair orgasmic response. Certain medical conditions such as spinal cord injury, multiple sclerosis, hormone conditions and diabetes have been implicated. Treatment of anorgasmia is often facilitated by a sex counselor or sex therapist with an emphasis on the couples developing playful and/or relaxed interactions. Success with therapy ranges from 65 to 85%.

73. What is Peyronie's disease and what causes it?

Peyronie's disease is a benign condition of the penis that tends to affect middle-aged males. The exact cause of Peyronie's disease is not known. The disease is characterized by the formation of plaques in the tunica albuginea of the penis. These plaques may be felt on penile examination and at times can feel as hard as bone. The plaques are like scar tissue and affect the function of the tunica in that area. Because the plaque is not elastic and stretchy like the rest of the tunica, it pulls the penis to the side of the plaque during an erection and may also cause **wasting/narrowing** at the site of the plaque. There may also be pain associated with an erection. Lastly, because the plaque does not behave like normal tunica, it may also cause erectile troubles. The plaque may occur anywhere along the penile shaft but is more commonly identified on the top (dorsal) surface of the penis. More than one plaque may be palpable. The hallmarks of Peyronie's disease are a palpable plaque (a hard spot along the shaft of the penis that one can feel when examining the penis), penile curvature, and a painful erection.

Wasting/ narrowing

An indentation in the penis.

The disease typically has a slow onset, and most men cannot identify a precipitating factor. It is thought that minor trauma during intercourse leads to minor tears in the tunica or rupture of small blood vessels. Bleeding and abnormal healing occurs after this injury and produces the plaque. In some men, there is a family history of Peyronie's disease, and 16 to 20% of men with

Peyronie's have a disease called Dupuytren's contractures. An increased incidence of arterial disease (30%) and diabetes with its associated small arterial disease (2.7–12%) has also been noted in men with Peyronie's disease.

The natural history of Peyronie's disease is variable. The disease is thought to have two phases: the acute phase, which usually lasts up to 18 months and is associated with pain, penile curvature, and plaque formation, and a more chronic phase, in which there is minimal or no pain, a palpable plaque, and residual penile curvature. Over time, the disease may progress in about 42% of men, improve in 13%, and remain the same in about 45%. In many cases, the disease produces few symptoms, the curvature does not prevent sexual performance, and there is no pain or associated erectile dysfunction. In such cases, reassurance that there is nothing bad going on is often all that is necessary.

Peyronie's disease is evaluated by history and physical examination. It is important to know if there are any problems with achieving adequate erections, whether or not the curvature prevents penetration and the location of the curvature. Sometimes the physician will ask you to take a picture of your penis when it is erect to assess the location and degree of curvature. Another option is for the doctor to inject a medication, prostaglandin E1, into the penis, which causes you to have an erection and to examine you at that time.

74. How is Peyronie's disease treated?

Most physicians recommend an initial conservative approach during the acute, inflammatory phase of Peyronie's disease, which can last from 6 to 18 months and is characterized by penile pain, curvature, and a palpable plaque. During this period, medical treatment options include oral therapy (Vitamin E, POTABA, Tamoxifen, Colchicine) and intralesional therapies (Verapamil, Interferon). None of these therapies are FDA approved for the treatment of Peyronie's disease, and there are limited well-designed studies evaluating their efficacy.

- Vitamin E—100 mg of Vitamin E three times a day for a minimum of 4 months. Vitamin E is an antioxidant, and it is thought that it decreases further plaque formation, although some studies suggest it is no more effective than placebo.
- Injectable verapamil—Although it has been used, it has not been shown to be better than placebo.
- POTABA (potassium para aminobenzoate)—POTABA is a member of the vitamin B complex and is believed to prevent fibrosis (scarring) from occurring through its effects on increased oxygen uptake by the tissues. It is rapidly excreted in the urine and as a result it needs to be taken frequently throughout the day, every 3 to 4 hours. The standard regimen is 12 grams/day, divided into 6 doses of four 500 mg tabs, for a total of 24 tabs per day. It is recommended that POTABA be used for 6 to 12 months.
- Cortisone injection—There are two agents that have been used, dexamethasone (decadron) in a dose of 0.2 to 0.4 mg injected directly into the plaque weekly for a course of 10 weeks, and triamcinolone hexacetonide (Aristospan) 2 mg injected into the lesion once every 6 weeks for a total of 6 injections.

Surgical intervention is reserved for those individuals whose Peyronie's disease fails to resolve/improve with conservative therapy. Criteria for surgical intervention include: severe penile curvature which prevents intercourse, stable and unchanged disease for at least 3 months, and severe penile shortening.

There are three main approaches to the surgical management of Peyronie's disease:

1. Shortening of the tunica albuginea (plication procedure or corporoplasty) on the contralateral corpora

2. Lengthening of the affected corpora by incision or excision of the plaque and placement of a graft

3. Placement of a penile prosthesis to straighten the penis and restore erectile function

75. What are the current treatment options available for ED?

There are a variety of options available for the treatment of ED, ranging from oral therapy (PDE-5 inhibitors), intraurethral suppository, injection therapy, and the vacuum device to surgical intervention, placement of a penile prosthesis. **Table 18** lists the currently available treatment options and they are discussed individually in greater detail in the following questions.

76. What if my testosterone level is low? What are the risks and benefits of testosterone therapy?

Hypogonadism is a condition in which low levels of testosterone are found in association with specific signs and symptoms, including decreased desire (libido) and sense of vitality, erectile dysfunction, decreased muscle mass and bone density, depression, and anemia. When hypogonadism occurs in an older male, it is referred to as andropause, or androgen deficiency of the aging male. Hypogonadism is estimated to affect 2 to 4 million men in the United States, and its incidence increases with age. Only about 5% of affected males are being treated.

Table 18 Treatment Options for Erectile Dysfunction

Rx	Administration	Dosing	Success Rate	Contraindications	Side Effects	Mechanisms of Action
Sildenafil	Oral: taken on demand 0.5–1.5 hr before intercourse, requires stimulation	25, 50, 100 mg, lower dose if > 65 yr, use newer protease inhibitors, erythromycin, ketoconazole with hepatic/renal failure; 78% pts prefer 100 mg. Use only once per 24 hr.	48–81%; varies with etiology of erectile dysfunction	Concomitant nitrate use, retinitis pigmentosa. When using concomitant alpha-blockers, pt should be on stable dose of alpha-blocker prior to starting sildenafil; start with 25 mg dose. Follow Princeton guidelines regarding use in CV pts.	HA in 16%, flushing in 10%, dyspepsia in 7%, visual disturbance in 3%, priapism uncommon. NAION (nonarteritic anterior ischemic optic neuropathy) and hearing loss have been reported in individuals taking PDE 5 inhibitors, but a causal relationship has not been identified. The risk factors for NAION are similar to those for ED, such as age > 50 yr, HT, increased cholesterol, and DM. Another risk factor is a small cup-to-disk ratio. Pts should be advised to seek medical attention in the event of a sudden loss of vision in one or both eyes. Hearing loss has also been reported in patients taking PDE-5 inhibitors. As with NAION, a causal relationship has not been established.	Phosphodiesterase type V inhibitor leads to increased cGMP, which stimulates cavernous small muscle relaxation.

Table 18 Treatment Options for Erectile Dysfunction (*Continued*)

Rx	Administration	Dosing	Success Rate	Contraindications	Side Effects	Mechanisms of Action
Cialis	Oral: taken on demand 2 hr before intercourse, requires stimulation	5 mg, 10 mg, 20 mg. Recommended starting dose in most pts is 10 mg. Start at 5 mg if moderate renal insufficiency, lower dose if on CYP 3A4 inhibitors. Cialis has a long half-life of 17–21 hr, which may provide for efficacy for up to 36 hr, however, may be taken once every 24 hr. 2.5 mg once daily recently approved.	62–77% success with penetration (SEP 2) and 50–64% success with maintaining erection (SEP 3)	Nitrates, retinitis pigmentosa; if using alpha-blockers, must be stable on alpha-blocker therapy and start with lowest dose of cialis. Follow Princeton guidelines regarding use in CV pts.	HA 11–15%, dyspepsia 4–10%, myalgia 1–3%, back pain 3–6%, flushing 2–3%. NAION—see sildenafil side effects. Hearing loss—see sildenafil side effects.	Phosphodiesterase type V inhibitor leads to increased cGMP, which stimulates cavernous small muscle relaxation.

(*Continued*)

Table 18 Treatment Options for Erectile Dysfunction (Continued)

Rx	Administration	Dosing	Success Rate	Contraindications	Side Effects	Mechanisms of Action
Vardenafil	Oral: taken on demand 25 minutes to 60 minutes before intercourse, requires stimulation	2.5 mg, 5 mg, 10 mg, 20 mg. Recommended starting dose in most pts is 10 mgs. Start at 5 mg in pts ≥ 65 yr, lower doses when concomitant use with CYP3A4 inhibitors.	Improvements in SEP 2 (ability to penetrate) of 75–80% (10–20 mg) compared to 52% with placebo and maintenance of erection SEP 3 of 64–65% (10–20 mg) compared to 32% placebo.	Nitrates, retinitis pigmentosa; if using alpha-blockers, must be stable on alpha-blocker therapy and start with lowest dose of Vardenafil. Follow Princeton guidelines regarding use in cardiovascular pts. May increase QTc interval and thus avoid use in individuals with congenital QT prolongation and those taking Class IA or III antiarrhythmics.	HA 15%, flushing 11%, dyspepsia 4%. NAION—see sildenafil side effects. Hearing loss—see sildenafil side effects.	Phosphodiesterase type V inhibitor leads to increased cGMP, which stimulates cavernous small muscle relaxation.
Intraurethral alprostadil	Small suppository placed into distal urethra via small applicator	125, 250, 500, 1000 µg. Use only once per 24 hr.	30–66% success rate (*NEJM* 1997; 336:1)	Hypersensitivity to PGE1, pregnant partner, predisposition to priapism (leukemia, multiple myeloma, sickle cell).	Pain (penile, urethral, testicular, perineal) in 33%, lowers blood pressure in 3%, priapism, vaginal irritation in 10%.	Absorbed through urethral mucosa and stimulates arterial dilation and flow.
Intracavernous injection therapy with alprostadil	Direct injection into lateral aspect of corpora cavernosa, alternating sides with each injection	5 µg to > 40 µg; dose depends on etiology of ED; test dose at 10 µg; if suspect neurologic disease, use 5µg test dose; use only once per 48–72 hr.	Average success rate 73% (*Int J Impot Res* 1994;6:149; *J Urol* 1988; 140:66)	Known hypersensitivity to alprostadil. Pts at risk for priapism. Pts at increased risk: those on anticoagulants and with Peyronie's dz.	Prolonged erections in 1.1–1.3%, corporal fibrosis in 2.7%, painful erection in 15–30%, hematoma, ecchymosis in 1.5%.	Alprostadil stimulates cavernous small muscle relaxation, causes modulation of adenyl cyclase, increase in cAMP and subsequent free Ca^{2+} conc.

(Continued)

Erectile Dysfunction (ED)

Table 18 Treatment Options for Erectile Dysfunction (*Continued*)

Rx	Administration	Dosing	Success Rate	Contraindications	Side Effects	Mechanisms of Action
Vacuum constriction device	Plastic cylinder with hand- or battery-operated pump and constricting bands.	N/A. Remove band within 30 min after application.	68–83% satisfaction rate	Use with caution in pts taking aspirin or anticoagulants.	Painful ejaculation: 3–16%, inability to ejaculate: 12–30%, petechiae of penis: 25–39%, numbness during erection: 5% (*J Urol* 1993;149:290; Spahn M, Manning M, Juenemann KP. Textbook of Erectile Dysfunction) Carson C, Kirby R, Goldstein I. Oxford: Isis Medical Media 1999.	Vacuum device creates negative pressure that pulls blood into corpora cavernosa; constriction band prolongs erection by decreasing corporal venous drainage.
Penile prosthesis	Surgically placed; models range from semirigid to inflatable.	N/A	> 90% satisfaction with inflatable prostheses (*J Urol* 1993; 150:1814; 1992;147:62)	Decreases penile length by 1 cm. Infection < 10%, diabetics at increased risk. Mechanical malfunction < 5% (*Urol Clin North Am* 1995;22:847). Erosion: increased risk in diabetics and spinal cord injury pts.	Requires counseling, preoperative.	Cylinders placed in corpora cavernosa provide penile rigidity; once placed, there is corporal fibrosis; if removed, remaining options less likely to work.

Source: Ellsworth P, Caldamone, A. *The Little Black Book of Urology,* 2nd ed. Sudbury, MA; Jones and Bartlett; 2007:181–189.

Despite the reported benefits of testosterone replacement therapy, including improvement in libido, bone density, muscle mass, body composition, mood, red blood cell count, and cognition, its use remains controversial.

Despite the reported benefits of testosterone replacement therapy, including improvement in libido, bone density, muscle mass, body composition, mood, red blood cell count, and cognition, its use remains controversial. There remain concerns regarding the risks of hormone therapy, particularly with respect to the risk of effects on the prostate, both benign and cancerous disease, as well as cardiovascular risks.

There is no definitive data to support that testosterone-replacement therapy increases cardiovascular risk. In fact, studies of testosterone replacement therapy have not demonstrated an increased incidence of cardiovascular disease or events such as myocardial infarction, stroke, or angina. Large scale placebo controlled long-term studies are needed to assess the long-term cardiovascular risks of testosterone therapy.

The data on the effects of testosterone replacement therapy on lipid profiles are inconsistent. Supraphysiologic (higher than normal) doses of androgens have been shown to decrease high-density lipoprotein (HDL) levels. However, when physiologic (normal) replacement doses of testosterone (both in the intramuscular and transdermal formulations) have been used, there appears to be no change or only a small decrease in HDL levels.

Higher levels of testosterone appear to stimulate erythropoiesis. It appears that injections are associated with a greater risk of erythrocytosis than topical preparations. In males receiving testosterone replacement therapy, the hematocrit or hemoglobin level should be monitored so that appropriate interventions, such as dose reduction, withholding of testosterone, therapeutic phlebotomy, or blood donation, may be performed if erythrocytosis occurs.

Testosterone replacement therapy has been associated with increases in prostate volume, primarily during the first 6 months of treatment. Despite the increase in size of the prostate there do not appear to be significant changes in voiding symptoms, urine flow rates, and postvoid residual volumes.

Controversy exists regarding the impact of testosterone replacement therapy on prostate cancer risk. Androgen ablation therapy remains one of the primary forms of therapy for metastatic prostate cancer. Despite the hormone responsiveness of prostate cancer there is no compelling data to associate the risk of developing prostate cancer with testosterone replacement therapy. There is also no compelling data to suggest that men with higher testosterone levels are at greater risk of prostate cancer or that treating men who have hypogonadism with supplemental testosterone therapy increases this risk. However, proper monitoring with measurement of PSA and digital rectal examination should promote the early diagnosis, thus potentially the cure, of most unmasked prostate cancers identified during testosterone treatment. The role of testosterone replacement therapy in hypogonadal men who have undergone curative treatment for prostate cancer is also controversial. Historically, it was felt that testosterone replacement therapy was contraindicated in men with a history of prostate cancer, but this is being challenged in the hypogonadal male who has been treated and cured of prostate cancer.

The currently used formulations of testosterone (intramuscular, gel, transbuccal, and patch) do not appear to have significant effects on liver function and routine monitoring of liver function is not necessary. Oral testosterone therapy, which is not FDA-approved in the United States, is associated with potential liver toxicity.

Testosterone replacement therapy has been associated with worsening of sleep apnea or with development of sleep apnea. This appears to be more common in men treated with intramuscular testosterone and who have other risk factors for sleep apnea.

Other reported adverse effects of testosterone therapy include: breast tenderness and swelling, decreased testicular size, adverse effects on fertility (particularly with the intramuscular formulation related to its high peaks), skin reactions (primarily erythema and pruritus) with transdermal formulations, pain and swelling at the site of injection for intramuscular testosterone, fluid retention which is usually mild in nature, but may be clinically significant in men with congestive heart failure, acne, oily skin, increased body hair, and flushing.

77. Are there different types of testosterone therapy?

There are several different types of available testosterone therapies (**Table 19**).

Oral Testosterone Therapy

Currently, oral testosterone therapy is not used in the United States. In other countries, an oral form of testosterone (testosterone undecenoate) is available that is well-tolerated and provides more consistent testosterone levels.

Parenteral (Intramuscular) Testosterone Therapy

Parenteral testosterone is inexpensive and safe, but has several disadvantages. Use of parenteral testosterone requires periodic deep intramuscular (IM, into the muscle) injections, usually every 2 to 3 weeks. Use of testosterone injection therapy results in supraphysiologic (higher than normal) levels of testosterone, usually

Table 19 Comparison of Testosterone Replacement Therapies

Type Of Therapy	Dose	Frequency	Side Effects	Cost
INJECTABLE				
Testosterone enanthate and Cypionate	100–400 mg	Q 1–4 weeks	• Supraphysiologic level 2–5 days after injection • Peak may be associated with breast tenderness, gynecomastia, and mood swings. • May affect spermatogenesis. • Highest incidence of side effects	Less expensive
Testosterone pellets		Q 6 months	• Risk of erythrocytosis • 8.5% risk of pellet extrusion	Expensive
TOPICAL THERAPY				
Androderm nonscrotal patch	12.2 mg patch delivers 2.5 mg/day; 24.3 patch delivers 5 mg/day	Daily	• 37% pruritis • 12% burn-like blisters • 0.1% triamcinolone cream under reservoir decreases incidence and severity of skin reactions	Less expensive
Testoderm TTS nonscrotal patch	328 mg patch delivers 5 mg/day	Daily	• 12% itching • 3% erythema	Less expensive
Testoderm scrotal patch	4 mg and 6 mg patch	Daily	• 7% itching • 4% discomfort • 2% irritation	Less expensive
Androgel 1% testosterone gel	5 g (50 mg), 7.5g (75 mg), 10 g (100 mg) packet	Daily	• 5.6% application site reaction	Expensive
Transbuccal	30 mg	BID	• Most closely mimics normal circadian rhythm • Gingival irritation	Very expensive

Reprinted from *Urologic Nursing*, 2008, Volume 28, Number 5, p. 366. Reprinted with permission of the publisher, the Society of Urologic Nurses and Associates, Inc. (SUNA), East Holly Avenue, Box 56, Pitman, NJ 08071-0056; (856) 256-2300; FAX (856) 589-7463; E-mail: uronsg@ajj.com; Web site: www.suna.org.

within 3 days of the shot. These levels steadily decline over the next 10–14 days, with a low level occurring around the time of the next injection. This peak-and-trough effect can affect one's mood, well-being, and sexual interest; in some men, these fluctuations can be disturbing. The risk of developing erythrocytosis (increased number of red blood cells) is 44% with injection therapy compared to only 3–18% with transdermal (gel or patch) therapy. Lastly, high peaks in testosterone levels are associated with negative effects on sperm production, so caution is warranted when treating men who are interested in having children with IM testosterone therapy. The recommended dose of intramuscular testosterone is 200–400 mg every 10–21 days to maintain normal average testosterone levels.

A long-acting form of testosterone, testosterone undecanoate (Nebido, Endo) is approved for use in Europe and is in clinical trials in the United States, awaiting evaluation by the FDA. With this formulation, patients typically require only about four injections per year of 1000 mg/4ml. An advantage of the long-acting formulation is less variability in testosterone levels. Side effects are the same as the other IM testosterone formulations. The two most common side effects are acne and discomfort at the injection site.

Transdermal Testosterone Therapy
Two forms of transdermal testosterone therapy are available: patch and gel.

Transdermal testosterone patch therapy (Testoderm, Testoderm TTS, and Androderm) provides one of the most physiologic restorations of testosterone level—meaning that the therapy brings your testosterone level back to levels resembling the natural amount of testosterone that should be in your body throughout the day. Transdermal testosterone therapy (therapy that enters through the skin) can be given as a scrotal patch or a nonscrotal patch. The limitations of the scrotal patch (Testoderm) make it less appealing: Its use requires shaving the scrotum—and in some men, the scrotum may be too small to apply the patch. The nonscrotal patch (Androderm, Testoderm TTS) must be applied to a nonhair-bearing skin surface and one to which pressure is not applied (i.e., you cannot put the patch on your buttocks because pressure would be applied when you sit down). Also, the site of patch placement must be rotated each day.

The testosterone patch is usually applied at bedtime and produces the highest testosterone level in the morning and the lowest level at the time of next patch application; this pattern matches the variation in testosterone levels normally seen over the course of a day. Unlike with the parenteral form of testosterone, the transdermal form has little effect on the blood cell count. The most common side effects of the patch are skin related and may vary from skin irritation to a chemical burn. Application of triamcinolone cream to the skin underneath the patch reservoir decreases the incidence of skin irritation.

The Androderm patch is available in 2.5 mg and 5 mg versions. The usual daily dose is 5 mg, but individual dosing will vary with testosterone levels. The skin patch achieves normal testosterone levels in 67 to 90% of men.

Another form of transdermal testosterone therapy is a topical gel applied to the skin (Androgel, Testim). Gel therapy produces normal testosterone levels in 87% of men. Androgel is available as a 5 g gel packet that delivers 5 mg of testosterone daily. The usual starting dose is 5 g, but the dose may be increased to 7.5 g or 10 g, depending on the individual's original serum testosterone levels. Testim is also a 5 g dose (the gel contains 50 mg of testosterone, but only 10% of it is delivered through the skin); its dose also may be increased to 10 g based on the individual's serum testosterone levels. A testosterone level is usually checked about 2 weeks after starting gel therapy.

Like the patch form of testosterone, the gel is applied once daily. Once applied, it is important to make sure that the gel has completely dried prior to wiping the affected area. You should not shower or swim shortly after the gel is applied. You must also be careful about physical contact when the gel is first applied because it may be absorbed by your partner if it gets onto your partner's skin. The gel therapy is easy to use and does not cause skin irritation, but it is more expensive than some other forms of testosterone therapy.

Buccal Therapy

Striant, a transbuccal form of testosterone therapy has been approved by the FDA. This buccal system contains 30 mg of testosterone and is used twice each day, in the morning and in the evening. This method of testosterone administration most closely mimics the normal daily variation in testosterone levels. Although Striant is easy to use, it may cause some gum irritation. In one study, 97% of men had a normal testosterone level when taking transbuccal therapy.

78. Do I need to be monitored while on testosterone therapy?

All hypogonadal men receiving testosterone replacement therapy require monitoring. All men should have a baseline PSA, hemoglobin level, and digital rectal examination prior to the start of testosterone replacement therapy. Those males with an elevated PSA and/or abnormal digital rectal examination should undergo further evaluation to rule out prostate cancer prior to starting testosterone replacement therapy. Once testosterone therapy has been started, patients return for an assessment of the efficacy of treatment and measurement of testosterone levels. Once an appropriate dose of testosterone has been identified, patients are followed at 3 to 6 month intervals during the first year and yearly thereafter. At each visit, an assessment of response, voiding symptoms, and sleep apnea symptoms should be determined. In addition, a digital rectal examination is performed and blood tests, including serum testosterone, PSA and hemoglobin/hematocrit levels. In patients receiving intramuscular testosterone, there is more variability in the serum testosterone levels. Typically, the testosterone levels peak 2 to 5 days after the injection and often return to baseline at 10 to 14 days after injection. This variability must be kept in mind when interpreting testosterone level results.

The PSA may also increase due to benign growth of the prostate over time. It is generally accepted that the PSA should not increase by 0.7 to 0.75 ng/ml per year and thus an increase in PSA beyond 0.35 ng/ml over a 6 month period would prompt withholding of the testosterone therapy and further evaluation with a transrectal ultrasound guided prostate biopsy. If the hemoglobin/hematocrit increases beyond the normal range, consideration should be given to withholding testosterone replacement therapy, reducing the dosage of testosterone, or if clinically significant and/or in high risk patients, performing a phlebotomy.

79. What is priapism and what causes it?

Priapism is a persistent abnormal erection of the penis, usually without sexual desire, and is accompanied by pain and tenderness. A lack of detumescence is referred to as a prolonged erection if the duration of the rigidity is fewer than 4–6 hours and priapism if the erection lasts longer than 4–6 hours. If the erection lasts longer than 6–8 hours, it is often associated with pain. Priapism may occur from too much blood flow into the penis (high flow), or it may be a result of too little blood flow out of the penis (low flow).

High-flow priapism may occur after there has been an injury to the penis that causes damage to an artery that results in unregulated blood flow into the penis. Because there is an increase in arterial blood (which carries oxygen) into the penis, high-flow priapism does not cause pain. In high-flow priapism, there is venous drainage out of the penis, so the erection does not tend to be as rigid as in a full erection.

Low-flow priapism occurs more in men with sickle cell disease/trait—a condition in which the red blood cells take on an abnormal (sickle) shape in response to decreased oxygenation, dehydration, and acidosis—and cancers of the blood, such as leukemia. It may also occur with injection therapy for erectile dysfunction and with certain psychiatric medications, such as trazodone. It has also been seen in men taking illicit drugs such as cocaine and marijuana. Because the problem consists of a problem with drainage of blood from the penis, which has little oxygen in it, this form of priapism is associated with pain and full rigidity.

The treatment of priapism varies with whether or not it is high flow or low flow and the duration of symptoms. The treatment of high-flow priapism focuses on stopping the inflow of blood through the abnormal artery. This can be achieved by injecting a chemical into the penis that tells the arteries to close down or by occluding the abnormal artery. Specialized radiologists are able to identify the abnormal artery and inject a substance or device into the artery to block it off. Because more than one artery supplies blood to the penis, this embolization does not usually cause any damage to the penis or to subsequent erections.

If treated early, low-flow priapism can be treated with the injection of a medication into the side of the penis. If the man waits too long and the rigidity has lasted longer than 6 hours, then a physician must first wash out the stagnant blood from the penis before injecting the chemical that stops the erectile process. In certain cases, surgical treatment is required to bring the erection down. Thus, if one has an erection that is continuing at 3 hours it is important to go to the emergency room. Early intervention with low-flow priapism is essential. Waiting too long can affect penile health and prevent responses to medications for ED in the future.

Early intervention with low-flow priapism is essential. Waiting too long can affect penile health and prevent responses to medications for ED in the future.

80. What are oral therapies for ED— specifically, the phosphodiesterase type 5 (PDE-5) inhibitors?

Currently, three oral therapies are available for the treatment of ED. The first therapy to become available was sildenafil (Pfizer's Viagra), which was approved by the FDA in 1998. Vardenafil (Bayer's Levitra) and tadalafil (Lily Icos's Cialis) were approved for use years later. All three of these oral therapies are phosphodiesterase type 5 (PDE-5) inhibitors.

To understand how these therapies work, it is important to review the process involved in the normal erection. When aroused or stimulated sexually, the brain sends messages from nerves in the pelvis, resulting in the release of nitric oxide. The nitric oxide then stimulates the production of cGMP, which in turn tells the cavernosal muscle in the penis to relax, thereby allowing more blood to flow into the penis. cGMP is broken down in the penis by an enzyme, phosphodiesterase type 5 (PDE-5) (**Figure 32**). Thus, if PDE-5 is prevented from working by administration of a PDE-5 inhibitor, there will be more cGMP present and thus a greater stimulus for increased blood flow.

Critical to the success of all of the PDE-5 inhibitors is the need for sexual arousal (sexual stimulation) after taking the medication. That is, these medications will not cause an erection to occur without sexual stimulation. It is okay to have a glass of wine, a beer, or a mixed drink when using these therapies—such limited alcohol consumption should not interfere with their effectiveness. Too much alcohol, however, may have a negative effect on erectile function, so a man should limit his alcohol intake when taking any of these medications.

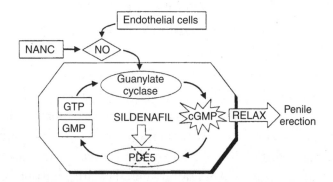

Figure 32   **Neurologic mechanism of erectile function. Sexual stimulation leads to release of nitric oxide, which leads to an increase in cGMP, a neurotransmitter that causes smooth muscle relaxation and increased blood flow into the penis. Abbreviations within the figure are: cGMP, cyclic guanosine monophosphate; GMP, guanosine monophosphate; GTP, guanosine triphosphate; NANC, nonadrenergic-noncholinergic neurons; CO, nitric oxide; PDES, phosphodiesterase type 5.**

Reprinted with permission from *Am J Cardiol* 1999; 84(5B):11N–17N.

81. Who is a candidate for oral therapy with a PDE-5 inhibitor?

Most men can take PDE-5 inhibitors. Nevertheless, there are certain contraindications to the use of these therapies. If these limitations are ignored, serious or even life-threatening problems may occur.

Specific contraindications to the use of PDE-5 inhibitors include the use of products containing organic nitrates, such as sublingual nitroglycerin, amyl nitrates, nitro-glycerin patches, and long-acting nitrates such as Imdur (**Table 20**). Nitrates (e.g., nitroglycerin), which are a form of nitric acid that causes opening of the blood vessels to the heart, and nitrites should not be used for angina for at least 24 hours after a man has taken a PDE-5 inhibitor.

Table 20   Commonly Prescribed Nitrates

Brand Name (Various)	
Cardilate	Nitrogard
Cartrax	Nitroglyri
Deponit (transdermal)	Nitrolingual Spray
Dilitrate & Dilitrate SR	Nitrol Ointment (Appli-Kit)
Duotrate	Nitrong
Imdur	Nitropar
Iso-Bid	Nitropress
Iso-D	Nitrostat
Isordil	Nitro-Time
Isotrate	Onset-5
Isrno	Papavatral
Miltrate & Miltrate 10	Pennate
Minitran Transdermal System	Penta Cap #1
Monoket	Pentrate
Nitrek	Pentritol
Nitro-Bid	Peritrate
Nitrocin (sustained release)	Sorbide-lO
Nitrocine	Sorbitrate & Sorbitrate SR
Nitrocot	Tetrate-30
Nitro-Derm	Transderm-Nitro
Nitrodisc	Transdermal NTG
Nitro-Dur	Tridil

Source: Ellsworth, P. *100 Questions and Answers About Erectile Dysfunction, 2e.* Jones and Bartlett Publishers, LLC, 2008.

When combined, nitrates and PDE-5 inhibitors may significantly lower blood pressure to a potentially life-threatening level. For this reason, a contradiction to the use of PDE-5 inhibitors is unstable angina requiring frequent use of short-acting or sublingual nitroglycerin.

Should you experience chest pain during intercourse, you should stop what you are doing. If the pain persists, you should go to the emergency room and notify the personnel there that you took a PDE-5 inhibitor so that they will know not to give you any form of nitrate.

The use of PDE-5 inhibitors has not been studied in patients with the following conditions, so caution should be used in treating such individuals with a PDE-5 inhibitor: congestive heart failure with a borderline low blood volume, recent heart attack (myocardial infarction), hypotension (low blood pressure), high blood pressure requiring 3 or more medications, retinitis pigmentosa (a congenital eye condition that causes blindness), severe arrhythmias (irregular heartbeat), and any condition that may make men prone to priapism such as sickle cell disease/trait, leukemia, and multiple myeloma.

If you are unsure of your cardiac status, you have a strong family history of cardiovascular disease, or you do not exercise regularly, then you should consider seeking further cardiac evaluation before you begin using a PDE-5 inhibitor. A cardiac stress test can help determine whether you have any significant cardiac risks associated with sex and the use of a PDE-5 inhibitor.

Males taking alpha-blockers, doxazosin (Cardura), terazosin (Hytrin), tamsulosin (Flowmax), and silodosin (Rapaflo) should be on stable doses of the alpha-blocker prior to starting PDE-5 therapy and should start at the lowest dose of the PDE-5 inhibitor. Although

PDE-5 inhibitors cause minimal effects on blood pressure, when used in conjunction with the alpha-blockers, which also may lower the blood pressure, the result may be clinically significant, so it is best to be cautious and follow the dosing guidelines.

How do I use PDE-5 inhibitors?

Use of PDE-5 inhibitors is on demand, meaning that in most cases, each time you want to have intercourse, you need to take a pill. These pills facilitate your body's response, rather than causing an erection on their own, so they require sexual stimulation or foreplay to work. Other medications that increase PDE-5 inhibitor levels include erythromycin (E-mycin), clarithromycin (Biaxin), ketoconazole (Nizoral), itraconazole (Sporanox), and cimetidine (Tagamet). Men taking protease inhibitors, such as indinavir (Crixivan), nelfinavir (Viracept), ritonavir (Norvir), or saquinavir (Fortovase), should start at a lower dose and take the PDE-5 inhibitor less frequently because the protease inhibitors (generally prescribed for HIV infection and AIDS) increase the blood levels of the PDE-5 inhibitors.

The three PDE-5 inhibitors vary somewhat in terms of how far in advance a man needs to take the medication for it to be effective and how long after taking the medication he can anticipate a response. Both sildenafil (Viagra) and vardenafil (Levitra) should be taken about 1 hour prior to intercourse, whereas tadalafil (Cialis) should be taken 2 hours prior to anticipated intercourse. Diet may affect the results with sildenafil—specifically, an individual should avoid consuming a high-fat meal prior to using this drug. Tadalafil has a long half-life (17–21 hours); thus, if this medication works for you, it may work for as long as 3 days after you initially take the medication. This is not the case for all men. Recently, a lower dose of tadalafil has been approved for daily use.

Multiple doses are available for each of these medications, but it is recommended that you start at the lowest dose and titrate the dose upward as needed. In certain patients, a lower dose and less frequent use of the medication are recommended. Your doctor will tell you which dose and dosing interval is appropriate for you. All of the PDE-5 inhibitors should be taken only once in a 24-hour period.

82. What is the success rate for PDE-5 inhibitors?

Overall, the PDE-5 inhibitors have a similar success rate. Success rates range from 48 to 81% with the various therapies, depending on the etiology of the ED. Individuals who have failed to respond to one of these medications may, however, respond to a different PDE-5 inhibitor. In one study, vardenafil was shown to be helpful in patients who had previously failed to respond to sildenafil therapy. However, studies have also demonstrated that patients who have failed an initial trial of sildenafil, when educated regarding proper use and rechallenged with sildenafil, have an increased likelihood of responding. Similarly, if you experience bothersome side effects with one medication, let your doctor know and your doctor may recommend trying a different PDE-5 inhibitor.

In men who have External-Beam Radiation Therapy-related erectile dysfunction, response rates range from 48 to 90%.

The response to PDE-5 inhibitors post-radical prostatectomy vary with several factors including patient's erectile status prior to the surgery and nerve-sparing status. The success rates of sildenafil for men who have undergone a bilateral nerve-sparing radical prostatectomy are approximately 70%; for those who have undergone a unilateral nerve-sparing radical prostatectomy, they are approximately 50%; and for those who have undergone a non–nerve-sparing radical prostatectomy, the success rates are approximately 15%.

PDE-5 inhibitors have been shown to be quite effective in reversing antidepressant-induced sexual dysfunction and antipsychotic-induced sexual dysfunction.

83. What are the side effects of PDE-5 inhibitors?

Several side effects are associated with all three of the currently available PDE-5 inhibitors—namely, headache, flushing, nasal congestion, and dyspepsia. Headache, flushing, and nasal congestion are vasodilatory effects and reflect dilation (increased opening) of blood vessels in the head, face, skin of the chest, and nasal mucosa, respectively. Dyspepsia (indigestion) may occur as a result of relaxation of the gastroesophageal sphincter. The gastroesophageal sphincter lies at the junction between the stomach and the esophagus (the tube through which food passes to enter into the stomach after you swallow). With relaxation of the sphincter, reflux (back-flow) of acidic stomach contents into the esophagus may occur, causing a sour taste.

The abnormal vision that can occur with sildenafil use typically involves a change in color vision (abnormal blue/green discrimination) related to the inhibitory effect of sildenafil on phosphodiesterase type 6 in the eye. This visual disturbance is not reported in patients taking tadalafil or vardenafil (Levitra). Myalgia has been reported in 1–3% of men taking tadalafil, however, though this effect is usually responsive to nonsteroidal anti-inflammatory medications such as ibuprofen.

All three of the currently marketed PDE-5 inhibitors may cause mild, transient decreases in blood pressure. In most cases, such elevations do not cause any side effects. In men who take multiple medications for high blood pressure or those with low blood pressure (hypotension), however, even this mild change in blood pressure may be significant. Similarly, men who take alpha blockers for benign prostate enlargement (BPH) are cautioned about taking PDE-5 inhibitors.

Since the FDA's approval of sildenafil, tadalafil, and vardenafil, a few rare side effects have been reported with these medications. Although none of these side effects is necessarily caused by the PDE-5 inhibitor, patients and doctors should still be aware of the following:

- Heart attacks and death. In some cases, these cardiac events are clearly related to the combined use of nitroglycerin-containing products and a PDE-5 inhibitor. Some such events have occurred in men with known cardiovascular disease, but other patients who experienced these problems have not had previously identified cardiovascular disease. Given this fact, men with cardiovascular disease should discuss the risks of PDE-5 inhibitor use with their primary care provider or cardiologist (if they have one) prior to taking the PDE-5 inhibitor. If you are unsure about the status of your cardiovascular health, you should discuss the possibility of further evaluation, such as a stress test, with your primary care provider.
- Stroke.

- Onset of irregular fast heartbeat (atrial fibrillation).
- Priapism. This side effect has been reported on rare occasions with use of PDE-5 inhibitors. If you experience an erection lasting 2 to 3 hours, it is important that you seek immediate care. Failure to obtain treatment in a timely fashion could potentially cause further penile damage.
- Nonarteritic ischemic optic neuropathy (NAION) has been reported with all three PDE-5 inhibitors since they entered the market and were used in larger groups of patients than had participated in the clinical trials of these drugs. NAION is a sudden, painless loss of vision, which may affect one or both eyes. At this time, a cause-and-effect relationship between PDE-5 inhibitor use and NAION has not been established. Several medical conditions that cause erectile dysfunction are also risk factors for NAION, including hypertension, diabetes mellitus, atherosclerosis, and elevated cholesterol. Another condition, crowded disc, also increases the risk of NAION. If you experience a sudden loss of vision when taking a PDE-5 inhibitor, it is recommended that you seek medical attention immediately. A large study that evaluated 52,000 patient over years of observations revealed that the incidence of NAION in men taking sildenafil was similar to that reported in the general population. A causal relationship between PDE-5 inhibitor use and NAION has not been demonstrated, however, because of the temporal relationship between PDE-5 inhibitor use and NAOIN, it is recommended that patients be warned of this side effect and to stop using the medication if they experience symptoms and contact their doctor.
- Hearing loss has been reported with all three PDE-5 inhibitors since they entered the market. A temporal

relationship between use of a PDE-5 inhibitor and loss of hearing has been noted, but a cause-and-effect relationship between PDE-5 inhibitor use and loss of hearing has not been established. As with NAOIN, underlying medical conditions in the patients may have contributed to the hearing loss, the numbers are too small to draw any formal conclusions. The FDA has recommended that physicians should advise patients to stop taking PDE-5 inhibitors and seek prompt medical attention in the event of sudden decrease or loss of hearing. The loss of hearing may be accompanied by tinnitus and dizziness.

84. What is intraurethral alprostadil (MUSE) and how do I use it?

Intraurethral alprostadil (Vivus's MUSE) is an intraurethral medication (i.e., a drug that is injected into the urethra) that was approved by the FDA in June 1998. Alprostadil is a synthetic form of a normal body chemical, prostaglandin E_1, that causes increased blood flow into the penis. MUSE works differently than sildenafil (Viagra), the oral therapy for ED. That is, the prostaglandin in MUSE stimulates the production of a chemical called cAMP, which, like cGMP, can cause the relaxation of smooth muscle and thus increase blood flow to the penis.

MUSE is an on-demand medication, meaning that you must take it each time that you wish to achieve an erection. The suppository of the alprostadil is enclosed in a small applicator (**Figure 33**). You should void before inserting the tip of the applicator into your penis, because voiding helps lubricate the urethra. Other topical lubricants, such as K-Y Jelly, Vaseline, and mineral oil, cannot be used with MUSE because they interfere with the absorption of the alprostadil. Once the applicator

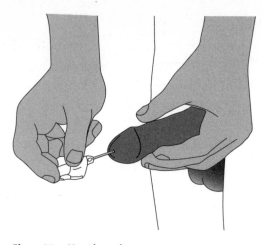

Figure 33   Muse insertion.

is placed into the urethra, you squeeze the small round button at the end, which releases the suppository into the urethra. Gently rocking the applicator from side to side will ensure that the suppository disengages from the applicator and remains within the urethra when the applicator is removed. Once the applicator is removed, gentle massaging of the penis causes the suppository to dissolve in the urethra.

Once in the penis, the alprostadil is absorbed through the urethral tissue and travels via blood vessels into the corpora cavernosa (the erectile tissue of the penis). There, it stimulates dilation of the arteries and provides for relaxation of the cavernosal smooth muscle within 10 to 20 minutes. The onset of a response to the MUSE is quick, usually occurring within 7 to 20 minutes after it is administered. The duration of the response varies with the dose and ranges from 60 to 80 minutes.

Several doses of MUSE are available: 125, 250, 500, and 1000 µg. This medication must be refrigerated.

85. Who is a candidate for MUSE?

There are relatively few contraindications to the use of MUSE. Because MUSE is administered intraurethrally and not all of the dose may be absorbed at the time of ejaculation, you should not use this therapy if your partner is pregnant.

Men who have undergone prior radical prostatectomy appear to have an increased risk of penile or urethral burning with MUSE, and they should be warned about this possibility. The exact cause of this side effect is not known, but it may be caused by a postsurgical supersensitivity of the corpora or increased retention of the MUSE in the penis because the dorsal vein may have been tied off at the time of radical prostatectomy. In particular, patients who have experienced pain with alprostadil in the past are likely to experience discomfort with MUSE. Hypotension (low blood pressure) and syncope (fainting) have been noted with MUSE as well and can be associated with serious cardiovascular consequences. For this reason, MUSE should be used with caution in men who have significant cardiovascular risks and in older men. In addition, the use of MUSE requires test dosing in the office to ensure that there is no hypotensive or syncopal event with use. Men who are at increased risk for priapism, such as those with sickle cell anemia, leukemia, polycythemia, thrombocythemia, or multiple myeloma, should not use MUSE. Men in whom sexual activity is not advisable, such as those with severe cardiovascular disease, should not use MUSE.

86. What is the success rate of MUSE?

In the initial studies of MUSE's effectiveness, the success rate was 64%. More recent studies have demonstrated its efficacy to be only 30%, however. Attempts to increase this success rate via the use of the ACTIS venous constrictor, a constricting band that is placed at the base of the penis, have helped some men. In some men, an erection rigid enough for penetration may occur in the standing position; however, when these individuals change to a supine position, the erection may decrease. In these men, changing the position used for intercourse or using the constricting band has proved helpful.

It is difficult to predict who will and who will not respond to MUSE. The patient's age and the cause of the erectile dysfunction, for example, are not predictive of response. Nevertheless, MUSE is unlikely to be effective in men who have not responded to intracavernous injection therapy.

MUSE is unlikely to be effective in men who have not responded to intracavernous injection therapy.

87. What are the side effects of MUSE?

The most common side effect, occurring in one-third to one-half of all men who take MUSE, is pain. This pain may be present in the penis, urethra, testis, or perineum. The intensity of the pain varies according to the dose taken. Thus, as the dose increases, the intensity of the pain may likewise increase. Hypotension and syncopal episodes (temporary loss of consciousness caused by decreased blood flow to the brain) have been reported in 1.2 to 4% of men who took MUSE, with their frequency depending on the dose used. Other side effects include urethral bleeding (in 4 to 5% of men who took MUSE), dizziness (in 1%), and urinary tract infection (in 0.2%). Prolonged erections and penile fibrosis (scarring) rarely occur. Ten percent of female partners experience vaginal irritation or vaginitis.

88. What is penile injection therapy?

Intracavernous injection therapy is the process whereby a small amount of a chemical is injected directly into the corpora cavernosa. These chemicals relax smooth muscle, thereby helping to increase blood flow into the penis.

The major advantage of injection therapy is that it does not depend on oral absorption, as pills do, or on absorption through the tissues, as MUSE does. The disadvantage is that it requires a small penile injection. Most men are anxious when they initially start with injection therapy but find that the procedure itself is not especially uncomfortable. In most patients who do not respond to first-line oral therapy or who are not candidates for oral therapy, injection therapy provides satisfactory erections.

The only FDA-approved chemicals for intracavernous injection therapy are Caverject (Pharmacia & Upjohn) and Edex (Schwarz Pharma) (Table 21). Both of these agents consist of prostaglandin E_1. Other agents used alone or in combination include papaverine and phentolamine. All three medications—prostaglandin E_1, papaverine, and phentolamine—may be used in combination, in which case the combination is referred to as triple P or trimix. Prostaglandin E_1 and triple P are the two most common forms of injection therapy used, and each offers a unique set of advantages and disadvantages.

How do I perform penile injection therapy?

Before you start to use intracavernous injection therapy at home, you will receive a test dose in the physician's office. Of all of the therapies available, intracavernous injection therapy carries the highest risk of priapism, with as many as 2% of patients experiencing this side effect. Most cases of priapism occur with first use, during the test dosing. This fact is important because if you return to your urologist's office within 3–4 hours, the erection can easily be brought back down with an injection of another chemical. If your urologist is concerned about priapism, he or she may choose to terminate your erection by injecting you with a chemical to stop the erection before you head home. Thus, test dosing minimizes your risk of having a case of priapism at an inopportune time.

Your urologist can also use the test dosing session as a time for hands-on instruction. That is, you can learn how to inject yourself and actually perform your first self-injection with the physician's guidance in the office. This consideration is very important because the first time you perform the injection therapy at home, you will probably be nervous. Remembering that you performed the injection in the office may help you relax.

The needle that you use to inject the medication is quite short and small. It is short because it does not need to pierce deeply into the penis, just into the corpora on one side, for the therapy to be effective (**Figure 34**). It is small because you will be injecting only 1 cc or less

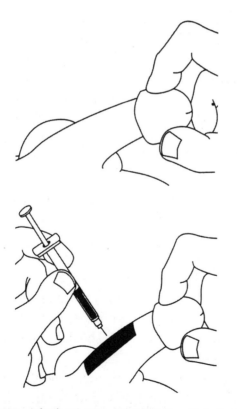

Figure 34   Injection therapy: Proper location of injection.

Used with permission from Pfizer, Inc.

Table 21   Dosage and Volume Calculations for Injection Therapy Using Prostaglandin E$_1$ (Caverject, Edex)

10 µg/mL vial	Dose Volume 20 µg/mL vial	40 µg/mL vial
1.0 µg/0.10 mL	2.5 µg/0.125 mL	10 µg/0.25 mL
2.0 µg/0.20 mL	5.0 µg/0.25 mL	16 µg/0.40 mL
2.5 µg/0.25 mL	7.5 µg/0.375 mL	20 µg/0.50 mL
5.0 µg/0.50 mL	10.0 µg/0.50 mL	24 µg/0.6 mL
7.5 µg/0.75 mL	15.0 µg/0.75 mL	30 µg/0.75 mL
10.0 µg/1.0 mL	20 µg/1.0 mL	40 µg/1.0 mL

Source: Ellsworth, P. *100 Questions and Answers About Erectile Dysfunction, 2e.* Jones and Bartlett Publishers, LLC, 2008.

of medication. After your initial test dose, your urologist will decide on a dose that you will try initially at home. The volume you inject will vary with the amount of prostaglandin E$_1$ you need to achieve an adequate erection and the concentration of the solution (**Table 21**). Do not get discouraged if this initial dose is not adequate. Most physicians would prefer to prescribe a dose that is too small and then increase it as needed to avoid priapism.

When using injection therapy at home, you should keep several points in mind:

- Look where you are going to inject the syringe to make sure that no superficial veins are in the area.
- Gently wipe the area with an alcohol swab.
- Always inject the medication on the side of the penis toward the base. The needle should be inserted straight into the penis at a 90-degree angle to the penis.
- Apply pressure to the injection site for a minute or two. If you see any bleeding from the injection site, maintain the pressure for about 5 minutes. Men taking

blood thinners should apply pressure to the injection site for about 5 minutes.

- Never reinject the medication once you have made the initial injection, even if you fear that you have not injected yourself properly.
- Alternate sides with each injection.
- Do not inject medication more frequently than every 48–72 hours.
- If your erection lasts longer than 3 hours, call the urologist on call. Do not wait—a delay in seeking care will just make it more difficult to treat the prolonged erection.
- If you are having difficulty with performing the injections, talk with your urologist. Perhaps getting more instruction or an autoinjector (e.g., the PenInject 2.25 autoinjector) or teaching your partner would be helpful.
- Remember that with Edex and Caverject, once the medication has been reconstituted (i.e., once the powder is dissolved in the sterile water), it must be refrigerated. The solutions tend to lose their efficacy after 7 days.
- Make sure that the volume of the medication and the dose of medication that you are injecting are consistent (see the calculations in Table 21).
- Do not reuse needles and carefully dispose of used needles.
- Remember that your erection may persist after you climax and ejaculate, but will go down when the medication wears off and exits from your system.

Bob's comment:

Some people resolve their erectile dysfunction through the use of injection therapy—I was, but am no longer, a member of that group. Because I am an insulin-dependent diabetic, I have had much experience with needles. Twice daily, I use an insulin-laden syringe to satiate my body's need to control my sugar levels. There is one big difference between injection therapy for erectile dysfunction and insulin injections for diabetes: With diabetes I inject my arms, legs, or abdomen; with the injection therapy for erectile dysfunction, I inject my penis. To me, that is a big difference.

I was first introduced to injection therapy as a quick means to achieve an erection. The physician primed what seemed to me to be a rather large syringe with the fluid, that, when injected, would cause an erection. I was instructed that this was accomplished by injecting the needle into the side of my penis. Within minutes, voila, an errection!

Needless to say, I was not overly excited when the instructions and test-doing were performed in the office, and I was less enthralled when I self-injected at home. In fact, after the first success in the physician's office, subsequent injections at home produced erections that were less firm and ineffective. Upon discussion with my physician, the dosage was increased. However, as we continued to go up and up on the medication, it just didn't seem to improve things. Maybe the problem was related to my diabetes or maybe it was my mind— hard to say. Perhaps the injection itself was my undoing. Preparing for a sexual interlude, I would isolate myself in the bathroom, prepare the syringe, and then administer the injection. How romantic! Many an evening when the atmosphere was ripe for sex, I discretely (at least I thought I was being discreet) avoided the encounter. Envisioning the syringe and the prep was too much for me. No sale: I preferred to watch the Red Sox.

89. Who is a candidate for penile injection therapy?

Because the injection requires manual dexterity, it is important that the man be able to perform self-injection.

In some men for whom giving an injection may be difficult or who are anxious about pushing the needle into the side of their penis, an autoinjector is available that makes this task easier. Another option is to have the man's partner perform the injection. Similarly, if the man is obese and has trouble seeing his penis, self-injection may be difficult, so he would need to enlist the aid of his partner.

If a man has tried MUSE in the past and has experienced significant discomfort with it, then using Caverject or Edex will merely cause further discomfort. In this situation, it would be more appropriate to try triple P. In addition, if the man has a known hypersensitivity or has had a prior reaction to prostaglandins, then Caverject or Edex would not be appropriate. Depending on the severity of the reaction, however, the man might consider using bimix (papaverine and phentolamine only).

In a number of conditions, injection therapy may potentially produce additional side effects. For example, men who are prone to priapism, such as those with sickle cell disease or trait, multiple myeloma, and leukemia, are at increased risk for priapism if they use injection therapy. Men with Peyronie's disease should be aware that the process of injection causes local trauma to the tunica albuginea, which could theoretically cause new plaques to form. Men who are taking blood thinners, such as warfarin (Coumadin), can use injection therapy, but should apply pressure to the injection site for a minute or so to prevent a bruise. Men who are taking a monoamine oxidase inhibitor (an older type of antidepressant), such as Marplan, Nardil, Phenelzine, or Parnate, should not use this therapy.

90. What is the success rate of penile injection therapy?

Success rates for intracavernous injection therapy range from 70–94%. This kind of treatment is helpful in ED of all causes. Although injection therapy does not interfere with orgasm or ejaculation, its long-term success requires that the individual be comfortable with the injection process. Besides its overall success rate, another advantage of injection therapy is its quick onset of action, within 5 to 20 minutes of injection.

The dose required to achieve a successful erection varies greatly with the cause of the erectile dysfunction. Young men with spinal cord injury may require only 1 µg of Caverject or Edex, whereas older men with vascular disease and diabetes may require 40 µg of these medications.

91. What are the risks of penile injection therapy?

Despite the high efficacy and relatively benign side-effect profile of injection therapy, there is a high discontinuation rate with this treatment for ED. A recent review demonstrated that 15% of men who are offered injection therapy do not even try it, 40% discontinue treatment within 3 months, and only 20–30% of men continue with injection therapy for more than 3 years. Reasons for discontinuation include fear of needles, the injected volume, adverse effects, partner discontent with this mode of therapy, loss of partner or relationship issues, problems with the ability to administer the medication, and the return of spontaneous erections. Other side effects include: (1) pain—injection site-related or diffuse, (2) hematoma—increased risk in men taking blood thinners, (3) priapism, (4) penile fibrosis—scar tissue within the corpora which may lead to a need for a higher dose of medication, (5) plaque formation—palpable scar tissue at the site of needle penetration of the corpora. The risk of liver injury with injection therapy is low and does not appear to be a concern for men using Caverject or Edex.

92. What is the vacuum device?

The vacuum device is a safe, reliable, reversible, noninvasive method of achieving an erection.

The function of the device is based on two principles:

1. A vacuum, or negative pressure, is generated to pull blood into the penis.
2. A constriction device (ring) is used at the base of the penis to decrease venous drainage and thus prolong the erection.

The vacuum device consists of a plastic cylinder, a pump that is either battery or hand operated, and one or more constrictive bands (**Figure 35**). The cylinder is wide enough and long enough to accommodate the erect penis. It is closed at the tip and open at the base. The constrictive bands are preloaded onto the base of the cylinder before its use.

How do I use the vacuum device?

To use the vacuum device, the constricting band is first placed onto the base of the cylinder, and the cylinder is then placed over the penis and pressed firmly against the pubic bone to achieve an airtight seal (Figure 35). Suction is applied by either a battery- or hand-operated pump. When the penis is rigid, the band is slipped off the cylinder and onto the base of the penis.

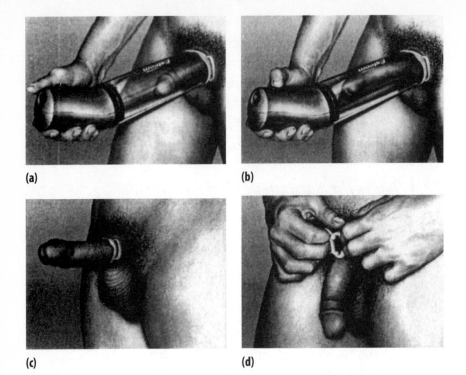

(a)   (b)

(c)   (d)

Figure 35   The vacuum device: (a) The vacuum deivce's pump creates a suction that pulls blood into the penis. (b) Within minutes, a nearly natural erection is produced. (c) A band is placed at the base of the penis to hold blood in the penis. (d) The constructing band is removed after intercourse. It should not be left on for more than 30 minutes.

Reprinted with permission from Timm Medical Technologies, Inc.

When intercourse is finished, the band is removed, and the blood drains out of the penis.

The time taken to achieve an erection with the vacuum device varies but may be as short as 2–3 minutes. The band may be left on the penis for 30 minutes only. Most men are able to quickly learn how to use the device and become comfortable with using it within four practice sessions.

Bob's comment:

I have tried the vacuum device but never had much satisfaction with it. For me, the preparation and the mechanics of achieving and sustaining an erection with the device were too much. I was dubious right from the onset, when the vacuum device's manufacturer's representative met with me in the doctor's office to demonstrate the device. He unveiled a 10-inch cylindrical container that was placed over my flaccid penis after I had affixed some Mason jar-type rubber rings at the base of the device. After the vacuum device has created an erection, I would have to dislodge these rings from the base of the device so that they were around the base of my penis. The rings would then squeeze the base of my penis to maintain the erection.

My skepticism started the day that the representative showed me the device and assited me with a live demonstration, at which time I asked myself, "Who designed this thing?" In fact, I really questioned why the representative would want this job—surely there were other career opportunities that he found more appealing. My skepticism persisted because despite the arduous presexual preparation, the vacuum device just never worked adequately for me. The rubber rings didn't seem to be sufficiently tight to maintain the erection. I will say, however, that of all of the other therapies that I tried before the placement of a penial prosthesis, the vacuum device did produce the firmest erection.

Perhaps it was my attitude; maybe it was my physiology. However, even though I used the vacuum device a score of times over a year or so, I knew that this was not for me over the long term. The romanticism and the spontaneity of sex were not there with the vacuum device.

93. Who is a candidate for the vacuum device?

Most men may use the vacuum device, and there are relatively few contraindications to its use. Men who have bleeding problems or who are taking blood thinners can use the vacuum device but must be careful. Men with Peyronie's disease who have significant penile curvature may not be able to use the device because the erect penis may not fit in the cylinder. In such cases, corrective surgery to straighten the penis may be performed before the use of the vacuum device, or the man can try using the device and generating a less rigid erection. An uncooperative partner precludes the successful use of the device.

94. What are the success and satisfaction rates for the vacuum device?

The initial report on the vacuum device, which was published in 1985, reported a 90% success rate for this device in achieving an erection that was adequate for sexual performance. Since then, published success rates with the vacuum device have ranged from 84–95%, and overall satisfaction rates reported for this device have ranged from 72–94%. Notably, the vacuum device has been shown to be effective in treating men with erectile dysfunction of many different causes. In patients with spinal cord injuries, the success rate is reported to be 92%. In those with psychogenic erectile dysfunction, this device also yields good results. In men who have erectile dysfunction caused by arterial disease or after radical prostatectomy, the success rate ranges from 90–100%. Furthermore, the vacuum device is successful in some men who were impotent after the removal of a penile prosthesis.

Approximately 50–70% of individuals continue to use the vacuum device over the long term. Reasons for discontinuation of this therapy include issues unrelated to the device (e.g., return of spontaneous erections, loss of libido, or loss of partner), which were cited in 43% of cases in one study. In 57% of cases, the reason for discontinuation is related to side effects of the device or partner dissatisfaction.

Several studies have compared the vacuum device with other forms of treatment for ED. In a study of men who were using the vacuum device successfully and then tried sildenafil (Viagra), approximately one-third preferred to resume use of the vacuum device rather than continue with the oral medication, citing the fact that the vacuum device gave them a better-quality erection. In a study that compared intracavernosal therapy (injection therapy) with the vacuum device, there was a trend among younger patients who had a shorter period of ED to favor intracavernosal therapy.

Bob's comment:

I did not have very good results with this device. However, many users have achieved excellent results with this technology.

95. What are the side effects of the vacuum device?

Side effects of the vacuum device include the following:

- Penile coolness. With the vacuum device, penile skin temperature may decrease by 18°C.
- Penile skin cyanosis. Congestion outside the corpora may make the penile skin look blue. This problem resolves with removal of the constricting band.
- Increased girth. The penile width after use of the vacuum device is actually wider than is seen with a normal erection.
- Pain. The most common complaint, pain usually occurs when men first use the device. It may be related to either the vacuum or the constricting band. Discomfort during suction is noted in 20–40% of men who use the vacuum device, primarily in men who are just learning to use the device. The pain appears to decrease with continued use of the vacuum

device and may be related to initial unfamiliarity with the device. As many as 45% of men have pain at the site of the constricting band. Again, this discomfort seems to improve with time and familiarity with the device.

- Ejaculatory troubles. Pain with ejaculation is reported by 3–15% of men who use the vacuum device, and inability to ejaculate occurs in 12–30%.
- Penile bruising. This side effect is noted in 6–20% of men who use the vacuum device.
- Numbness during erection. This side effect occurs in 5% of men who use the vacuum device.
- Partner dissatisfaction. This rate ranges from 6–11%, with the following reasons for dissatisfaction being cited: unhappy with the performance, penile temperature, and penile appearance.

Severe complications (serious, undesired results of a treatment) are uncommon with use of the vacuum device, but they can occur. In particular, ischemia (decreased blood flow) of the penis leading to necrosis can occur if the constricting band is left on too long. This complication is more of a problem in men with spinal cord injuries because they do not feel the discomfort related to the band. If the band is removed within 30 minutes of application, the risk of penile ischemia is rare.

96. What is a penile prosthesis?

A penile prosthesis is an artificial device that, when placed in the penis, allows a man to have an erection. The development and use of penile prostheses began in the 1970s. Since then, numerous revisions and modifications in the prostheses have improved the satisfaction rate and mechanical durability of these devices.

The most commonly used is the three-piece prosthesis, which is comprised of two cylinders, a scrotal pump, and a separate reservoir that is placed in the pelvis (**Figure 36**). The advantage of the three-piece unit is that it allows for the maximal amount of fluid transfer given the larger reservoir size. Also, when placed correctly, the device and its tubing are completely concealed, so one is able to void in the locker room without anyone knowing that the multipart prosthesis is present. Multipart inflatable prostheses are made by American Medical Systems. Semirigid prostheses, although less popular, have less risk of mechanical problems (**Figure 37**). The semirigid prosthesis does not change in size, rather one simply bends the penis up or down for participation in intercourse.

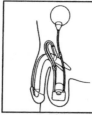 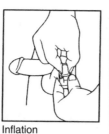 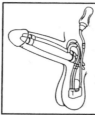 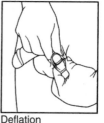

| Placement in body | Inflation | Erect state | Deflation |

Figure 36   Three-piece penile prosthesis.

Drawing of AMS 700CX™/CKM™ Penile Prosthesis courtesy of American Medical Systems, Inc., Minnetonka, MN (www.visitAMS.com).

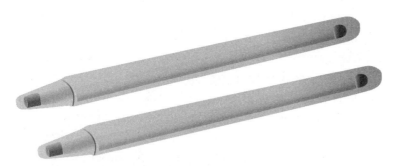

Figure 37   One piece, semi-rigid penile prosthesis.

Placement of a penile prosthesis requires extensive patient and partner discussion. It is not considered a first-line therapy in most cases of ED, but is an appropriate therapy for well-counseled individuals who have not responded to other therapies or who have found those alternatives to be unsatisfactory.

97. Who is a candidate for a penile prosthesis?

Penile prostheses are usually placed in men with organic ED. In men with psychogenic erectile dysfunction, extensive counseling should be administered and other treatment options should be exhausted before a penile prosthesis is considered. For all other patients, extensive patient and partner counseling should take place before placement of a prosthesis; the expectations, indications, and risks need to be discussed clearly, as well as other currently available and future options.

A penile prosthesis is rarely the first-line therapy for ED. In my practice, when I discuss penile prostheses with patients, I equate the procedure for its surgical placement with crossing over a rickety bridge that collapses once the prosthesis is implanted. You cannot go backward once the prosthesis is placed; if it is removed because of infection, malfunction, or dissatisfaction, other options of treatment are unlikely to work. Although there have been reports of the vacuum device and injection therapy working in some individuals after removal of a prosthesis, these instances are not common. For all these reasons, it is best to try all available therapies and determine whether they are successful and satisfactory before placement of a prosthesis occurs.

Indications for a penile prosthesis include the following:

- The patient's unwillingness to consider, failure to respond to, or inability to continue with other forms of treatment, such as oral therapy, injection therapy, MUSE, and the vacuum device
- Postinjection therapy penile fibrosis
- Peyronie's disease and erectile dysfunction
- Postpriapism erectile dysfunction
- Sex-change operations in women who undergo surgical creation of a penis
- Penile amputations in men, who then undergo surgical creation of a penis
- Psychogenic erectile dysfunction, after extensive counseling and evaluation
- Neurogenic bladders requiring condom catheters for urinary drainage

98. How do I use the penile prosthesis, and how is it placed?

Placement of a penile prosthesis is a surgical procedure that can be performed under general anesthesia or spinal anesthesia. You will stay in the hospital overnight and are usually able to go home the following morning.

To minimize the risk of infection, prior to the procedure your scrotal area is shaved, you are scrubbed with an antibacterial soap and you are given intravenous antibiotics to kill any residual bacteria that may be present on your skin. These intravenous antibiotics will be continued during your entire hospital stay, and you are discharged to home with a 10- to 14-day supply of oral antibiotics.

Three approaches to placement of the penile prosthesis are used, and the location of the incision varies with the type of prosthesis being placed and your surgeon's preference:

1. A subcoronal incision, a circumcision-type incision, is used for placement of semirigid prostheses.

2. A penoscrotal incision is used for placement of multipart prostheses, for reoperations, and in cases of penile fibrosis (scarring). This kind of incision is made in the midline of the upper part of the scrotum. If you look at your scrotum, you will see that a line runs up the middle of the scrotum; the incision is made in this line so that when it heals, it will be incorporated in the normal scrotal line.

3. Some surgeons use an infrapubic incision for placement of multipart prostheses. This kind of incision is made below the pubic bone near the base of the penis.

Usually, all components of a multipart prosthesis can be placed through a single incision. In some patients, prior abdominal and groin surgery—such as a hernia repair or a radical prostatectomy—may make placement of the reservoir of the three-piece prosthesis difficult. In this situation, your surgeon may make another incision on your abdomen to enable the reservoir to be implanted correctly. Each corpora cavernosa is opened and dilated to accommodate the cylinder. Each corpora is then measured. Your penis is actually much longer than you think—it extends back behind your pubic bone—and it is very important that the correct size of cylinder be placed. The pump is implanted either in the midline of your scrotum between the two testicles or on one side of the scrotum. You should discuss pump placement with your surgeon before surgery to ensure that its location will be easy for you to maneuver, particularly if you do not have good use of both hands. The reservoir in the three-piece unit is placed in the pelvis near the bladder. The tubing that connects the reservoir, pump, and cylinders runs deep under your skin so that it is not visible; if you feel closely, you may be able to identify the tubing, but the goal is to have it be unnoticeable. Before the procedure is completed, your surgeon will test the prosthesis to ensure that all components are working well, that when inflated it gives you a fully rigid erection, and that the tips of the prosthesis are in a good position in the tip of your penis.

Before the incision is closed, a small drain is placed to prevent a hematoma from forming, and the prosthesis is deflated. The surgeon may leave the prosthesis partially inflated and then deflate it the following morning because it can sometimes help prevent bleeding. When you wake up from surgery in the recovery room, you will have a catheter in place that drains your urine; a dressing around your penis, which will be taped up against your abdomen; and a drain in place.

In men with ED and prostate cancer who are undergoing a radical prostatectomy for treatment of their prostate cancer, the prosthesis can be placed at the time of surgery. There does not appear to be an increased risk of infection when this route is taken.

Bob's comment:

[I had my penile prosthesis] placed under general anesthesia. As a part of the initial discussion on the penile prothesis, Dr. Ellsworth discussed the mechanics of the prosthesis with me. As she was explaining the mechanics of the prosthesis, she must have noticed a puzzled look on my part. She said, "Do you want to see one?" "Sure," I responded. She returned carrying a rubbery device that has a manually operated pump at one end with two tentacles approximately

7 or 8 inches long protruding from either side. Frankly, it reminded me of one of those Day-Glo plastic Halloween skeletons that bobble all over the place. I said (to myself this time), "Is that thing going into my body?" It was. Incidentally, Dr. Ellsworth urged me to take the device home (in a brown paper bag) to show my wife and familiarize ourselves with the device.

After placement of the prosthesis and my hospital stay . . . I wanted nothing to do with activating the device for the first 3–4 weeks because of soreness in the vicinity of the incision. During this time, Dr. Ellsworth examined me periodically to ensure that there were no signs of a bacterial infection. Finally, when the tenderness had abated, the time came for Dr. Ellsworth to demonstrate how the penile prosthesis worked. The pump—the part that produces the erection—is inside the scrotum. It is somewhat rectangular in shape, about the size of a caramel candy, with a ball-type pump affixed on one side and the release valves along either end of the device. In principle, it works this way: Before intercourse, one locates the pump and presses it six or seven times to transfer fluid from the reservoir into the penile cylinders to create an erection. The penis will remain rigid as long as one desires. When one is finished with intercourse, one squeezes the release valves, and the fluid drains out of the cylinders and back into the reservoir. Gentle squeezing on the penis helps to get all of the fluid out of the cylinders. As with anything new, it is difficult to use initially, but with practice, it becomes much easier to use. It is not long before you adapt. It merely becomes part of you.

99. What are the risks of a penile prosthesis?

As with any surgical procedure, there are complications associated with the placement of a penile prosthesis. These risks may be subdivided into intraoperative complications (those occurring during surgery) and postoperative complications (those occurring after surgery).

Intraoperative Complications

Perforation

During dilation of the corpora cavernosa, the dilating instrument can perforate the urethra. If this occurs, the procedure must be terminated, the catheter must be left in place, and the urethra must be allowed to heal. If one cylinder has already been placed on the other side, it may be left in place and connected to the pump and reservoir before the surgery is completed. If the patient desires, the surgeon can go back in a few months and try to replace the cylinder. Some men find that they are able to achieve adequate rigidity with only one cylinder in place and do not wish to undergo another surgical procedure.

Similarly, during dilation of the corpora, a hole may be made from one corpus cavernosum into the other. The surgery can continue in this case, but the cylinders must be properly placed in each corpus cavernosum. If a hole is made, a cylinder may cross over, meaning that it starts in one corpus cavernosum but passes through the hole and ends in the other corpus cavernosum. If this situation goes unrecognized, it may cause asymmetry and pain with use of the prosthesis.

Existing Scarring

In individuals with significant penile fibrosis, such severe scarring may be present that narrower cylinders will be required. Rarely, it will be difficult to close the corpora over the cylinders. A patch of synthetic material or tissue must be removed from another area of your body in this case and used to cover the corporal defect.

Excessive Bleeding and Anesthesia Complications

As with all surgical procedures, there are bleeding and anesthetic risks with the implantation of a penile prosthesis.

Postoperative Complications

Decreased Penile Length

Decreased penile length is actually not a complication of penile implantation, but rather is intrinsic to the surgery. The cylinders are of a fixed length. To obtain penile rigidity, the cylinders increase in width (girth). Very observant patients will note a 1- to 2-cm decrease in penile length after the procedure.

Infection

One of the most devastating complications of penile prosthesis surgery is infection. Infection rates range from 2–16% in first-time procedures but increase to 8–18% in reoperations. Patients with diabetes and spinal cord injury, in particular, are at increased risk for infection.

Signs of infection include persistent pain, erosion of a part of the prosthesis, purulent drainage, fever, swelling and redness of the scrotum, and fixation of the tubing to the scrotal skin. In most cases, but particularly when infection occurs early after implantation, the entire prosthesis must be removed emergently. The area must then be irrigated with antibiotics, and intravenous antibiotics followed by oral antibiotics must be given. Implantation of a second prosthesis can be attempted 6 months later, after the area has completely healed.

When an infection occurs later and is caused by less aggressive bacteria, the surgeon may try to salvage the prosthesis. In such a case, the patient is taken to the operating room, the infected prosthesis is removed, the area is irrigated copiously with antibiotic solutions, and a new prosthesis is placed. The risk of infection associated with the new prosthesis in this situation is about 15%.

In an attempt to help decrease the risk of infection, some of the penile prostheses come impregnated with antibiotics and others have a coating which allows an antibiotic to be adhered to it.

Erosion and Migration

Erosion (destruction of a tissue surface) and migration (spontaneous change of place) of the prosthesis occur more commonly with placement of rigid prostheses and in men with indwelling catheters or on clean intermittent catheterization. These complications may also occur when the prosthesis is too long or the patient has an unsuspected urethral injury.

In the case of urethral erosion, there may be some splaying of the urine stream and the tip of the prosthesis may protrude into the urethra. In such cases, the affected cylinder is removed, and the corpora are irrigated with an antibiotic solution and closed. A catheter is placed into the bladder for about 1 week to promote urethral healing. A new cylinder can be placed 6 months later.

The tubing may also erode through the skin. Such tubing erosion is often a sign of a smoldering infection, in which case the best thing to do is to remove the prosthesis. The surgeon can also attempt the salvage technique described earlier.

Lastly, the cylinders may migrate proximally toward the base of the penis, a condition that shows up as a new droop in the glans. When this happens, the cylinder must be removed, the defect in the corpus cavernosum corrected, and the cylinder replaced.

Glans Droop

If the cylinders to be implanted are too short, they will not provide adequate support to the tip of the penis, causing the glans to droop. This drooping of the glans may make it difficult for the man to achieve vaginal penetration. A glans droop can be corrected by a simple surgical procedure and often does not require replacement of the prosthesis.

Penile Ischemia and Necrosis

These complications, which are extremely rare, occur when there is an injury to the blood supply to the corpora cavernosa or to the glans. Men with severe diabetes, those with extensive vascular disease, and those who require an extensive dissection for placement of the prosthesis are at increased risk of developing penile ischemia or necrosis. If the postoperative dressing is too tight, it may also cause ischemia.

Perineal Pain

Patients often experience some discomfort during the first 2 months or so after placement of a penile prosthesis. If the pain persists for a longer period, your physician may evaluate whether you have an infection or whether the prosthesis is too large. Some men may experience penile discomfort with the initial inflation of the prosthesis that is related to stretching of the tunica (the thick white membrane wrapped around the corpora cavernosa), but this usually resolves with time as the tunica stretches.

Residual Penile Curvature

In patients with Peyronie's disease, placement of the prosthesis and maneuvering of the prosthesis when it is erect in the operating room are usually all that is needed to correct the penile curvature that can occur with this condition. In rare cases, residual curvature may persist after placement of the prosthesis. If this condition does not improve with use of the prosthesis, then another procedure may be performed to excise the plaque.

Mechanical Problems

The incidence of mechanical problems with prostheses is approximately 5%—quite a low rate. Such problems may potentially include leaks, aneurysms, and rupture of the cylinders.

Leaks typically occur at connection sites and where the cylinder tubing enters the cylinder. Leaking prostheses either will not work or will not provide adequate rigidity. Connection site leaks may be easily repaired. A leaking cylinder can be replaced, but it is recommended that the entire prosthesis be replaced if the prosthesis has been implanted for a few years.

Aneurysms (i.e., dilations of a part of the cylinder) are very uncommon with the current prosthesis models. If they occur, the affected cylinder must be removed and replaced with a new device.

The cylinders can also rupture, usually as a result of unrecognized damage during the closure of the corpora. This problem is often detected when the device is inflated 4 to 6 weeks after surgery.

Autoinflation

Autoinflation is the phenomenon whereby the device inflates on its own without you manipulating the pump. It is the result of increased pressure around the reservoir. The newer penile prostheses have "lockout valves" which prevent autoinflation.

100. Is there a role for sex therapy in the treatment of ED?

Yes, there is often a role for sex therapy in the treatment of ED. You do not have to have psychogenic ED to potentially benefit from sex therapy. Sexual problems do not occur in isolation, nor are their effects limited only to the sexual arena. Sexual problems can be associated with relationship difficulties, decreased self-esteem, anxiety, and depression.

Sex therapy is very effective in helping people understand both the physiologic and the psychological aspects of ED. It also helps people identify and deal with unrealistic expectations and negative self-images, understand their partner's sexual needs and requirements, and dispel any myths about sexuality and sexual function that the patient and his partner may have. It also allows for help with relationship issues, such as intimacy conflicts, power and control struggles, and trust issues, which may be just as important as treatment of the ED in the restoration of a healthy sexual relationship.

Your doctor can help you locate a sex therapist in your area. A sex therapist may be a psychologist or psychiatrist who has a special interest in sexual dysfunction.

International Index of Erectile Function (IIEF)

A Multidimensional Scale for Assessment of Erectile Dysfunction

These questions ask about the effects your erection problems have had on your sex life over the past 4 weeks. Please answer the following questions as honestly and clearly as possible. In answering these questions, the following definitions apply:

- Sexual activity includes intercourse, caressing, foreplay, and masturbation.
- Sexual intercourse is defined as vaginal penetration of the partner (you entered your partner).
- Sexual stimulation includes situations like foreplay with a partner, looking at erotic pictures, etc.
- Ejaculate is the ejection of semen from the penis (or the feeling of this).

1. **Over the past 4 weeks, how often were you able to get an erection during sexual activity? Please check one box only.**

    ☐ No sexual activity
    ☐ Almost always/always
    ☐ Most times (much more than half the time)
    ☐ Sometimes (about half the time)
    ☐ A few times (much less than half the time)
    ☐ Almost never/never

2. **Over the past 4 weeks, when you had erections with sexual stimulation, how often were your erections hard enough for penetration? Please check one box only.**

    ☐ No sexual activity
    ☐ Almost always/always
    ☐ Most times (much more than half the time)
    ☐ Sometimes (about half the time)
    ☐ A few times (much less than half the time)
    ☐ Almost never/never

The next three questions will ask about the erections you may have had during sexual intercourse.

3. **Over the past 4 weeks, when you attempted sexual intercourse, how often were you able to penetrate (enter) your partner? Please check one box only.**
   - ☐ Did not attempt intercourse
   - ☐ Almost always/always
   - ☐ Most times (much more than half the time)
   - ☐ Sometimes (about half the time)
   - ☐ A few times (much less than half the time)
   - ☐ Almost never/never

4. **Over the past 4 weeks, during sexual intercourse, how often were you able to maintain your erection after you had penetrated (entered) your partner? Please check one box only.**
   - ☐ Did not attempt intercourse
   - ☐ Almost always/always
   - ☐ Most times (much more than half the time)
   - ☐ Sometimes (about half the time)
   - ☐ A few times (much less than half the time)
   - ☐ Almost never/never

5. **Over the past 4 weeks, during sexual intercourse, how difficult was it to maintain your erection to completion of intercourse? Please check one box only.**
   - ☐ Did not attempt intercourse
   - ☐ Extremely difficult
   - ☐ Very difficult
   - ☐ Difficult
   - ☐ Slightly difficult
   - ☐ Not difficult

6. **Over the past 4 weeks, how many times have you attempted sexual intercourse? Please check one box only.**
   - ☐ No attempts
   - ☐ 1–2 attempts
   - ☐ 3–4 attempts
   - ☐ 5–6 attempts
   - ☐ 7–10 attempts
   - ☐ 11+ attempts

7. **Over the past 4 weeks, when you attempted sexual intercourse, how often was it satisfactory for you? Please check one box only.**

☐ Did not attempt intercourse
☐ Almost always/always
☐ Most times (much more than half the time)
☐ Sometimes (about half the time)
☐ A few times (much less than half the time)
☐ Almost never/never

8. **Over the past 4 weeks, how much have you enjoyed sexual intercourse? Please check one box only.**

☐ No intercourse
☐ Very highly enjoyable
☐ Highly enjoyable
☐ Fairly enjoyable
☐ Not very enjoyable
☐ No enjoyment

9. **Over the past 4 weeks, when you had sexual stimulation or intercourse, how often did you ejaculate? Please check one box only.**

☐ No sexual stimulation/intercourse
☐ Almost always/always
☐ Most times (much more than half the time)
☐ Sometimes (about half the time)
☐ A few times (much less than half the time)
☐ Almost never/never

10. **Over the past 4 weeks, when you had sexual stimulation or intercourse, how often did you have the feeling of orgasm (with or without ejaculation)? Please check one box only.**

☐ No sexual stimulation/intercourse
☐ Almost always/always
☐ Most times (much more than half the time)
☐ Sometimes (about half the time)
☐ A few times (much less than half the time)
☐ Almost never/never

The next two questions ask about sexual desire. Let's define sexual desire as a feeling that may include wanting to have a sexual experience (e.g., masturbation or intercourse), thinking about having sex, or feeling frustrated due to lack of sex.

11. **Over the past 4 weeks, how often have you felt sexual desire? Please check one box only.**

    ☐ Almost always/always
    ☐ Most times (much more than half the time)
    ☐ Sometimes (about half the time)
    ☐ A few times (much less than half the time)
    ☐ Almost never/never

12. **Over the past 4 weeks, how would you rate your level of sexual desire? Please check one box only.**

    ☐ Very high
    ☐ High
    ☐ Moderate
    ☐ Low
    ☐ Very low or none at all

13. **Over the past 4 weeks, how satisfied have you been with your overall sex life? Please check one box only.**

    ☐ Very satisfied
    ☐ Moderately satisfied
    ☐ About equally satisfied and dissatisfied
    ☐ Moderately dissatisfied
    ☐ Very dissatisfied

14. **Over the past 4 weeks, how satisfied have you been with your sexual relationship with your partner? Please check one box only.**

    ☐ Very satisfied
    ☐ Moderately satisfied
    ☐ About equally satisfied and dissatisfied
    ☐ Moderately dissatisfied
    ☐ Very dissatisfied

15. Over the past 4 weeks, how do you rate your confidence that you can get and keep your erection? Please check one box only.

☐ Very high
☐ High
☐ Moderate
☐ Low
☐ Very low or none at all

Patient Instructions

Sexual health is an important part of an individual's overall physical and emotional well-being. Erectile dysfunction, also known as impotence, is one type of very common medical condition that affects sexual health. Fortunately, there are many different treatment options for erectile dysfunction. This questionnaire is designed to help you and your doctor identify whether you are experiencing erectile dysfunction. If you are, you may choose to discuss treatment options with your doctor.

Each question has several possible responses. Circle the number of the response that best describes your own situation. Please be sure that you select one and only one response for each question.

Over the Past 6 Months

1. How do you rate your *confidence* that you could get and keep an erection?

2. When you had erections with sexual stimulation, *how often* were your erections hard enough for penetration (entering your partner)?

3. During sexual intercourse, *how often* were you able to maintain your erection after you had penetrated (entered) your partner?

4. During sexual intercourse, *how difficult* was it to maintain your erection after you had penetrated (entered) your partner?

5. When you attempted sexual intercourse, *how often* was it satisfactory for you?

SCORE_____

Add the numbers corresponding to questions 1–5. If your score is 21 or less, you may want to speak with your doctor.

Resources

Organizations

American Academy of Medical Acupuncture

www.medicalacupuncture.org
By Telephone: 323-937-5514
By Mail: AAMA, 4929 Wilshire Boulevard, Suite 428,
   Los Angeles, California 90010

American Cancer Society

www.cancer.org
By Telephone: 1-800-ACS-2345
By Mail: American Cancer Society National Home Office,
   1599 Clifton Road, Atlanta, GA 30329
American Cancer Society Man to Man Support Groups
www.cancer.org/docroot/CRI/content/

American Foundation for Urologic Disease/ Prostate Health Council

www.afud.org
By Telephone: 800-242-2383
By Mail: 300 West Pratt Street, Suite 401, Baltimore, MD 21201-2463

American Prostate Society

www.ameripros.org
By Telephone: 410-859-3735
By Fax: 410-850-0818
By Mail: 1340-F Charwood Rd, Hanover, MD 21076

American Society of Clinical Oncology

www.asco.org
By Telephone: 703-299-0150
By Mail: 1900 Duke Street, Suite 200, Alexandria, VA 22314

American Urological Association

www.AUAnet.org
- clinical guidelines for the management of locally confined prostate cancer 2007, patient guidelines 2008
- clinical guidelines—reductase inhibitors for prostate cancer chemoprevention
- clinical guidelines for erectile dysfunction 2005
- clinical guidelines for premature ejaculation 2004
- clinical guidelines for BPH 2003
- clinical guidelines for priapism 2003

American Urological Association

Health Policy Department
By Telephone: 410-223-4367
By Mail: 1120 North Charles Street, Baltimore, MD 21201

American Urological Association Foundation

www.auafoundation.org or www.urologyhealth.org
By Telephone: 410-689-3700
Toll Free Number (U.S. only): 1-866-RING AUA (1-866-746-4282)
Fax: 410-689-3800
By Mail: Patient Education, 1000 Corporate Boulevard, Linthicum, MD 21090

Cancer Care, Inc.

www.cancercare.org
By Telephone: 212-712-8400 (admin); 212-712-8080 (services)
By Mail: 275 7th Avenue, New York, NY 10001

Cancer Research Institute

www.cancerresearch.org
By Telephone: 1-800-99-CANCER (800-992-26237)
By Mail: Cancer Research Institute, 681 Fifth Avenue, New York, NY 10022

CaPcure (The Association for the Cure of Cancer of the Prostate)

www.capcure.org
By Telephone: 800-757-CURE or 310-458-2873
By Mail: 1250 4th Street, Santa Monica, CA 90401

Centers for Disease Control and Prevention (CDC)

www.cdc.gov
By Telephone: 404-639-3534
Toll Free Number: 800-311-3435
By Mail: Centers for Disease Control and Prevention,
1600 Clifton Rd., Atlanta, GA 30333

Department of Veterans Affairs

www.va.gov
By Telephone: 202-273-5400 (Washington, D.C. office)
Toll Free Number: 800-827-1000 (reaches local VA office)
By Mail: Veterans Health Association, 810 Vermont Ave., NW,
Washington, DC, 20420

Health Insurance Association of America (HIAA)

www.hiaa.org
By Telephone: 202-824-1600
By Mail: 555 13th Street NW, Suite 600,
East Washington, D.C. 20004-1109

Health Resources and Services Administration

Hill-Burton Program
www.hrsa.gov/osp/dfcr/about/aboutdiv.htm
By Telephone: 301-443-5656
Toll Free Number: 800-638-0742
800-492-0359 (if calling from the Maryland area)
By Mail: Health Resources and Services Administration,
U.S. Department of Health and Human Services, Parklawn
Building, 5600 Fishers Lane, Rockville, MD 20857

International Cancer Alliance (ICARE)

www.icare.org/icare
By Telephone: 800-ICARE-61 or 301-654-7933
By Fax: 201-654-8684
By Mail: 4853 Cordell Avenue, Suite 11, Bethesda, MD 20814

International Society of Impotence Research

Contact: Mrs. Marianne Mulder
By Telephone: +31-24-3613920
By Mail: University Hospital Nigmegen, Department of Urology,
P.O. Box 9101, 6500 HB Nijmegen, The Netherlands

National Cancer Institute

www.nci.nih.gov

By Telephone: 301-435-3848 (Public Information Office line)

By Mail: National Cancer Institute Public Information Office, Building 31, Room 10A31, 1 Center Drive, MSC 2580, Bethesda, Maryland 20892-2580

National Center for Complementary and Alternative Medicine

www.nccam.nih.gov

By Telephone: 1-888-644-6226

By Mail: NCCAM Clearinghouse, P.O. Box 7923, Gaithersburg, Maryland 20898

National Comprehensive Cancer Network

www.nccn.org

By Telephone: 888-909-NCCN (888-909-6226)

By Mail: National Comprehensive Cancer Network, 50 Huntingdon Pike, Suite 200, Rockledge, PA 19046

The Impotence Association

www.impotence.org.uk

By Mail: PO Box 10296, London SW17 9WH, United Kingdom

Prostate Cancer

Astra Zeneca Pharmaceuticals LP

www.prostateinfo.com

The Prostate Cancer Education Council

By Telephone: 800-813-HOPE, 212-302-2400

By Mail: 1180 Avenue of the Americas, New York, NY 10036

The Prostate Cancer Infolink

www.comed.com/prostate

By Mail: c/o CoMed Communications, Inc., 210 West Washington Square, Philadelphia, PA 19106

Prostate Cancer Research and Education Foundation (PC-REF)

www.prostatecancer.com
By Telephone: 619-287-8860
By Fax: 619-287-8890
By Mail: 6699 Alvaro Rd, Suite 2301, San Diego, CA 92120

Prostate Cancer Resource Network

www.pcrn.org
By Telephone: 800-915-1001 or 813-848-2494
By Fax: 813-847-1619
By Mail: P.O. Box 966, Newport Richey, FL 34656

Social Security Administration

Office of Public Inquiries
www.ssa.gov
By Telephone: 800-772-1213 or 800-325-0778 (TTY)
By Mail: Social Security Administration, Office of Public
   Inquiries, 6401 Security Blvd., Room 4-C-5 Annex,
   Baltimore, MD 21235-6401

United Seniors Health Cooperative (USHC)

www.unitedseniorshealth.org
By Telephone: 202-479-6973
Toll Free Number: 800-637-2604
By Mail: USHC, Suite 200, 409 Third St, SW,
   Washington, DC 20024

Prostate Cancer Support

Alabama

US TOO Group

Affiliation: Southeast Alabama Medical Center
Doctor's Building, SE Alabama Medical Center, 7th Floor,
   1108 Ross Clark Circle, Dothan, AL 36301
334-794-3216
Meets the first Thursday of each month at 7:00 PM

US TOO PC Survivor Support Group

389 Clubhouse Drive, #DD4,
  Gulf Shores, AL 36542, 334-968-1115
Meets the first Thursday of each month, except
  September

California

Prostate Cancer Support Group

Affiliation: Fountain Valley Regional Hospital
11250 Warner Avenue, East Tower Cafeteria,
  Fountain Valley, CA
714-966-8055

Prostate Cancer Survivor's Support Group

Affiliation: Washington Hospital
200 Mowry Avenue at Civic Center Drive, Freemont, CA
510-657-0759
Meets each third Thursday, 7:00 to 9:00 PM, co-ed

The Prostate Forum, Fullerton

1st Presbyterian Church, 838 N. Euclid, Fullerton, CA
714-607-9241
Meets the second Tuesday and the fourth Tuesday from
  11:00 AM to 3:00 PM and 6:00 to 9:00 PM

Prostate Cancer Support Group

Medical Library at Marin General Hospital
Greenbrae on Bon Air Road
415-459-4668
Meets each Tuesday evening from 7:00 to 8:30 PM

Palo Alto VA Prostate Support Group

VA Palo Alto Health Care System
Building 101 Auditorium (1st floor near chapel)
408-996-7582
Meets the third Tuesday of every month from
  11:00 AM to 12:30 PM

Redwood City Support Group

702 Marshall Street, Redwood City, CA
650-367-5998
Meets on the first Tuesday of every month from 2:00 to 3:30 PM

San Jose Prostate Cancer Support Group

Camden Lifetime Activity Center, 3369 Union Avenue
   (just North of Camden Avenue), San Jose, CA
408-559-8553
Meets every second Wednesday of the month
   from 12:30 to 2:30 PM

San Mateo Support Group

Mid-Peninsula Medical Arts Bldg., 1720 El Camino
   Real, Atrium Room, Burlingame
San Mateo, CA
650-572-9035
Meets on the third Thursday from 1:00 to 3:00 PM

Santa Barbara PC Support Group

Burntress Auditorium, Cancer Center of Santa Barbara,
   300 W. Pueblo, Santa Barbara, CA
806-682-7300 or 805-969-7166
Meets on the second and fourth Thursdays
   from 2:30 to 3:30 PM

Santa Clara County: African American Prostate Cancer Support Group

408-226-3947

Santa Cruz County Prostate Cancer Support Group

Affiliation: US TOO, ACS
Dominican Hospital, Katz Cancer Resource Center
Website: www.scprostate.org
831-724-6446
Meets on the last Tuesday of the month from 7:00 to 9:00 PM

UCSF Comprehensive Cancer Center

San Francisco, CA
415-885-3693
Meets on the second and fourth Wednesdays from 6:00 to 7:00 PM

Silicon Valley Prostate Cancer Support

2500 Grant Road, Mountain View
Basement of El Camino Hospital
Meets every first Thursday of the month from 7:00 to 9:00 PM

Simi Valley US TOO Prostate Cancer Support Group

Aspen Center, 2750 Sycamore Drive, Simi Valley, Simi Valley, CA
805-522-4782

Florida

Jupiter Hospital

Jupiter, FL
561-743-5069
Meets every second Wednesday of every month at 5:00 PM

Man to Man

Auditorium of Sarasota Memorial Hospital
1700 S. Tamiami Trail (Rt. 41), Sarasota, FL
941-378-5647
Meets every fourth Monday of month at 2:00 PM

Georgia

Prostate Support Association

Affiliation: Emory Healthcare
Emory Clinic, 1365 Clifton Road, B Building, 5th Floor Conference
   Room, Atlanta, GA
404-727-4328

Illinois

US TOO International, Inc.

www.ustoo.com
903 North York Rd, Suite 50, Hinsdale, IL 60521-2993
Telephone: 800-808-7866 or 630-323-1002
Fax: 630-323-1003

Man to Man/Side by Side

Affiliation: American Cancer Society
Diversified Health Care Services,
    510 West Park, Champaign, IL
217-352-3042
Meets the first Thursday from 7:00 to 8:30 PM

Indiana

Man to Man Education and Support Group

Affiliation: American Cancer Society, St. Vincent Hospital
Cooling Auditorium at St. Vincent Hospital. 2001 W. 86th St.,
    Indianapolis, IN
317-849-1022
Meets from 6:45 to 8:30 PM

Well County Man to Man

Affiliation: American Cancer Society, Man to Man
Wells County Council on Aging, 225 W. Water St.,
    Bluffton, IN 46714
260-824-2986
Meets every second Monday of each month from
    4:00 to 5:30 PM

Kansas

US TOO Chapter

Via Christi-St. Joseph Medical Center, East Campus,
    3600 E. Harry, Wichita, KS
316-943-8274
Meets every second Monday of each month

Louisiana

Robert D. Knepper Man to Man Group

Affiliation: America Cancer Society
May Bird Perkins Cancer Center, 4950 Essen Lane,
    Baton Rouge, LA
Meets the first Monday of each month from 7:00 to 9:00 PM

Maryland

Man to Man Worcester County

Atlantic General Health Center, Ocean Pines Offices,
  11107 Racetrack Road, Berlin, MD
410-208-9555
Meets the first Tuesday of each month from 7:00 to 8:30 PM

Suburban Hospital

Bethesda, MD
301-896-3939
Meets on the third Monday of the month from 7:00 to 8:30 PM
  in conference rooms 6 and 7

VFW Prostate Cancer Support Group of DelMarVa

821 E. William Street, Salisbury, MD
410-835-2850
Meets at VFW Post 194 on the second Tuesday of the month for
  lunch, 1:30 PM for meeting

Michigan

The Survivor's Association

Grand Rapids, MI
616-356-4349
Meets at 7:00 PM on the first Tuesday of each month from
  September to June

Prostate Support Group

West Michigan Cancer Center, 200 N. Park St., Kalamazoo, MI
800-999-9748
Meets monthly on the last Wednesday at 7:00 PM

New Mexico

Prostate Cancer Support Association of New Mexico, Inc. (PCSA of NM)

Bear Canyon Senior Center, 4645 Pitt NE,
  Albuquerque, NM 87108
505-254-7784
Meets on the first and third Saturdays of the month from
  12:30 to 2:30 PM

Belen Support Group

Affiliation: PCSA of NM
120 South 9th Street, Belen, NM
505-861-1013

Carlsbad Support

Affiliation: PCSA of NM
2522 West Pearse St., Carlsbad, New Mexico
505-885-1557

Grants Support Group

Affiliation: PCSA of NM
Cibola Senior Center, 1150 Elm Drive, Grants, NM
505-285-3922

Santa Fe Support Group

Affiliation: PCSA of NM
Meeting Location: Cancer Treatment Center of Santa Fe,
    455 St. Michaels Drive, Santa Fe, NM
505-466-4242

Socorro Support Group

Affiliation: PCSA of NM
Meeting Location: 1228 Hilton Place, Socorro, New Mexico
505-835-4766

New York

Man to Man

Affiliation: American Cancer Society
95 Schwenk Drive, Kingston, NY
845-331-8300 or 800-233-5049
General meeting on the third Tuesday from 4:30 to 6:00 PM,
    Hurley Reformed Church Hall

Malecare

New York City, NY
212-844-8369
Meetings in several locations for spouse/partners, gays,
    transgendered

Monday: Men only, 6:00 PM, St. Vincent's Hospital Cancer,
325 W. 15th

Tuesday: Men and Women, 5:30 PM, Lenox Hill Hospital,
100 E. 77th, Conference Room 1

Tuesday: Men only, 7:00 PM, Beth Israel Hospital,
10 Union Square East, 4th Flr.

Wednesday: Men and Women, 6:00 PM, New York Presbyterian
Hospital, 16 W 60th, Suite 470

US TOO

Affiliation: Memorial Sloan Kettering/New York Presbyterian-
Cornell Chapter

Memorial Sloan Kettering, Hoffman Auditorium,
1275 New York Avenue, New York City, NY

212-717-3527

Meets on the third Thursday from 6:00 to
7:00 PM for the lecture and 7:00 to 8:30 PM for
the small group

Cancer Care, Inc.

275 7th Avenue, New York, NY

212-712-6121

Meets every first and third Tuesdays of the month from
5:30 to 7:00 PM

Woodbury Long Island

Affiliation: Cancer Care of Long Island

20 Crossways Park North, Suite 110, Woodbury, NY

516-364-8130, ext. 106

North Carolina

Prostate Cancer Support of Lee County

Affiliations: Man to Man, US TOO

Enrichment Center, 1615 South Third Street,
Sanford, NC 27330

919-774-6685

Meets on the second Wednesday of the month from
11:00 AM to 12:30 PM

US TOO Prostate Cancer Support Group of Wake County

Rex Cancer Center, Raleigh, NC
919-772-1047
Meets the second Thursday of the month at 7:00 PM

US TOO Prostate Support Group

Presbyterian Hospital, Raleigh, NC
704-563-9028

Wake County Prostate Cancer Support Group

Affiliations: American Cancer Society, US TOO,
   Rex Hospital
Rex Center, Cancer Center Auditorium, 4420 Lake Boone Trail,
   Raleigh, NC
919-846-8442
Meets from 7:00 to 9:00 PM on the second Thursday of the
   month except for December, July, and August

Ohio

Cincinnati Wellness Center

4918 Cooper Road, Cincinnati, OH
513-791-4060 or 513-321-1693
Small groups for men and women meet on the second
   Wednesday from 7:00 to 9:00 PM

James CCC PC Support Group

James Comprehensive Cancer Center
The Ohio State University
614-293-5066, 614-293-4646, or 800-293-5066
Meets the last Wednesday of each month: months alternate,
   men only

Oklahoma

US TOO of Central Oklahoma

Affiliation: US TOO
Oklahoma City, OK
405-604-4298

Meets on the third Monday from 6:00 to 7:30 PM; alternates between Deaconess Hospital and Integris Baptist Medical. Call for meeting locations

Oregon

Florence Support Group

Affiliation: American Cancer Society
400 9th Street, Florence, OR
541-997-6626
Meets on the first Monday from 5:30 to 7:00 PM in Conference Room C, Peace Harbor Hospital

Texas

Amarillo PC Support Group

Meeting Location: Luby's Cafeteria on Coulter
Amarillo, TX
806-355-0806
Meets first Thursday of every third month from 6:00 to 8:00 PM

Dallas

A support group for gay men dealing with prostate cancer in the Dallas/Fort Worth/Mid-Cities area of North Texas
972-235-0257
Dallas, TX

Washington

Man to Man of Everett, WA

Affiliation: American Cancer Society
Meeting Location: Medical Building Colby Campus, 14th and Colby, Everett, WA
360-568-2548
Meets on the third Wednesday from 7:00 to 9:00 PM; men only

Canada

Montréal West Island PC Support Group

Sarto Desnoyers Community Center, 1335 Lake Shore Drive, Dorval, Québec
514-694-6412

Meets at 7:30 PM every fourth Thursday of the month except
July, August, and December

Owen Sound (Ontario) PC Support Group

Affiliations: CPCN and US TOO
Meeting Location: St. Andrews Presbyterian Church
519-371-4779
Meets on the third Wednesday from 7:00 to 9:00 PM

Ireland

Men Against Cancer (MAC)

Sponsored by the Irish Cancer Society
c/o Irish Cancer Society, 43/45
Northumberland Rd., Dublin 4
Toll-Free Telephone: 1-800-200-700
Website: www.cancer.ie/support/mac.php

Israel

You Are Not Alone (YANA)

Israeli Cancer Association, Building 5, Haifa, Israel
04-837-1733
Meets 6:00 PM on the last Thursday of every month,
companions invited, meetings in Hebrew

South Africa

Wynberg Western Cape

Prostate Cancer Support Action (PSA) Group
Affiliation: National Cancer Association of South Africa
Southern Cross Hospital, First Floor Seminar Room
(021) 788-6280
Meets last Thursday of the month
Meets on the first Wednesday of the month from 11:30 AM
to 1:00 PM

Web Sites with General Cancer Information

www.411Cancer.com
www.about.com (search on "cancer")
www.CancerLinks.org
www.CancerSource.com

CancerWiseTM/MD Anderson Cancer Center:
  www.cancerwise.org
National Cancer Institute's CancerNet Service:
  www.cancernet.nci.nih.gov/index.html

Web Sites with BPH Information

www.kidney.niddk.nih.gov/kudiseases/pubs/prostateenlargement/
www.uroxatral.com, supported by Sanofi Aventis
www.4flomax.com, supported by Astellas and Boehringer
  Ingelheim
http://health.nytimes.com/health/guides/diseases/enlarged-
  prostate/overview.html
www.greenlightforbph.com, supported by American Medical
  Systems
www.hsrd.research.va.gov/publications/esp/BPH-2007.pdf

Web Sites with ED Information

www.urohealth.org, supported by Abbott Laboratories
www.medformation.com, supported by Allina Hospitals & Clinics
www.menshealthforum.org.uk, sponsored by the UK Men's
  Health Forum
www.viagra.com, supported by Pfizer Inc.
www.caverject.com, supported by Pfizer Inc.
www.levitra.com/about.html, supported by Bayer and Glaxo
  Smith Kline
www.cialis.com, supported by Lilly
www.kidney.niddk.nih.gov/kudiseases/pubs/impotence/
www.nlm.nih.gov/medlineplus/erectiledysfunction.html

Web Pages on Specific Topics

Alternative Therapy

Information on acupuncture: www.medicalacupuncture.org
  (see American Academy for Medical Acupuncture)

Comprehensive web site about alternative therapies for cancer:
  www.healthy.net/asp/templates/center.asp?centerid=23

Chemotherapy

Online and in-person support groups for those going through
  high-dose chemotherapy:
  www.yana.org

Drug information for chemotherapy and hormonal therapy, including information on financial assistance: www.cancersupportivecare.com/pharmacy.html.

Clinical Trials

National Cancer Institute's CancerTrials site lists current clinical trials that have been reviewed by NCI.

Coping

National Coalition for Cancer Survivorship (www.cansearch.org, 877-NCCS-YES) offers a free audio program, "Cancer Survivor Toolbox", including ways to cope with the illness. (Web site also has a newsletter, requiring yearly membership fee.)

R.A. Bloch Cancer Foundation (www.blochcancer.org) offers an inspirational online book about cancer, relaxation techniques, and positive outlooks on fighting cancer, as well as trained one-on-one support from fellow cancer patients.

Diet and Nutrition (Cancer Prevention)

USDA Dietary Guidelines: www.usda.gov/cnpp

American Institute for Cancer Research provides tips on how to reduce cancer risk: www.aicr.org

Cancer Research Foundation of America's Healthy Eating Suggestions: www.preventcancer.org/whdiet.cfm

Family Resources

www.kidscope.org is a web site designed to help children understand and deal with the effects of cancer on a parent

Genetic Counseling

The National Society of Genetic Counselors web site (www.nsgc.org) lists society members, complete with specialty.

The National Cancer Institute has a searchable list of health care professionals who specialize in genetics and can provide information and counseling: http://cancernet.nci.nih.gov/genesrch.shtml

Articles on genetics and cancer: http://cancer.med.upenn.edu/causeprevent/genetics

Legal Protections, Financial Resources, and Insurance Coverage

The American Cancer Society offers a number of relevant documents to help understand your coverage, legal protections, and how to find financial assistance. Search www.cancer.org using keyword "insurance."

Medicaid Information:
www.hcfa.gov/medical/medicaid.htm

"Every Question You Need to Ask Before Selling Your Life Insurance Policy." National Viator Representatives, Inc. Call 800-932-0050 for a free copy.
Internet: www.nvrnvr.com

Family and Medical Leave Act:
www.dol.gov/dol/esa/public/regs/statutes/whd/fmla.htm

Health Care Financing Administration's (HCFA) information website about Breast Cancer and Medicaid programs:
www.hcfa.gov/medicaid/bccpt/default.htm

www.needymeds.com offers information about programs sponsored by pharmaceutical manufacturers to help people who cannot afford to purchase necessary drugs.

www.cancercare.org/hhrd/hhrd_financial.htm offers listings of where to look for financial assistance.

The National Financial Resource Book for Patients: A State-by-State Directory: www.data.patientadvocate.org/

Nausea/Vomiting

National Comprehensive Cancer Network:
www.nccn.org/patient_guidelines/nausea-and-vomiting/
nausea-and-vomiting/1_introduction.htm

Royal Marsden Hospital Patient Information On-Line:
www.royalmarsden.org/patientinfo/booklets/coping/nausea7.
asp#heading

Treatment Locators: Physicians and Hospitals

AIM DocFinder (*State Medical Board Executive Directors*):
www.docboard.org/
Nonprofit organization providing a health professional licensing database.

AMA Physician Select (*American Medical Association*):
www.amaassn.org/aps/amahg.htm
AMA database of demographic and professional information
on individual physicians in the United States.

American Board of Medical Specialties: provides verification of
physician qualifications and has lists of specialists.
www.abms.org/, 1-866-ASK-ABMS or American Board of
Medical Specialties, 1007 Church Street, Suite 404, Evanston,
IL 60201-5913

Best Hospitals Finder (*U.S. News & World Report*):
www.usnews.com/usnews/nycu/health/hosptl/tophosp.htm

The *U.S. News* hospital rankings are designed to assist patients in
their search for the highest level of medical care. Database is
searchable by specialty, including the top cancer hospitals
(www.usnews.com/usnews/nycu/health/hosptl/speccanc.htm)
or by geographic region.

Best HMOs Finder (*U.S. News & World Report*): *U.S. News*
guide to choosing a managed-care option:
www.usnews.com/usnews/nycu/health/hetophmo.htm

Hospital Select (*American Medical Association & Medical-Net, Inc.*):
www.hospitalselect.com/curb_db/owa/sp_hospselect.main
Hospital locator database searchable by hospital name, city,
state, or zip code. Hospital Select data include basic information (name, address, telephone number); beds and utilization;
service lines; and accreditation.

National Cancer Institute Designated Cancer Centers:
www.cancertrials.nci.nih.gov/finding/centers/html/map.html
Directory of NCI-designated Cancer Centers: 58 research-
oriented U.S. institutions recognized for scientific excellence
and extensive cancer resources. Listings feature phone contact
numbers, website links, and a brief summary of website resources.

National Comprehensive Cancer Network (NCCN):
www.nccn.org
The National Comprehensive Cancer Network (NCCN) is an
alliance of leading cancer centers. NCCN members
(www.nccn.org/profiles.htm) provide the highest quality in cancer
care and cancer research. NCCN offers a patient information
and referral service (www.nccn.org/newsletters/1999_may/

page_5.htm) that responds to cancer-related inquiries and provides referrals to member institutions' programs and services (1-888-909-6226).

Approved Hospital Cancer Program (*Commission on Cancer of the American College of Surgeons*):
www.facs.org/public_info/yourhealth/aahcp.html
The Approvals Program of the Commission on Cancer surveys hospitals, treatment centers, and other facilities according to standards set by the Committee on Approvals, which recommends approval awards in specific categories based on these surveys. A hospital that has received approval has voluntarily committed itself to providing the best in diagnosis and treatment of cancer. Approved hospitals can be searched by city, state, and category.

Association of Community Cancer Centers: Cancer Centers and Member Profiles:
www.accc-cancer.org/members/map.html
Geographic listing of ACCC members with contact information, and description of cancer program and services *as provided by the member institutions*.

HMOs and Other Managed Care Plans (Cancer Care):
www.cancercare.org/patients/hmos.htm
Discusses the advantages and disadvantages of HMO care.

Physician Qualifications

The American Board of Medical Specialities at: www.abms.org; click on "who's certified" button (search by physician name or by specialty)

Radiation Therapy

National Cancer Institute/CancerNet: Radiation Therapy and You: A Guide to Self-Help During Cancer Treatment at: www.cancernet.nci.nih.gov/peb/radiation/. By toll-free telephone: 1-800-4-CANCER (in English and Spanish)

Books and Pamphlets

The following pamphlets are available from the National Cancer Institute by calling 1-800-4-CANCER:

"Chemotherapy and You: A Guide to Self-Help During Treatment"

"Eating Hints for Cancer Patients Before, During, and After
Treatment"
"Get Relief From Cancer Pain"
"Helping Yourself During Chemotherapy"
"Questions and Answers About Pain Control: A Guide for
People with Cancer and Their Families"
"Taking Time: Support for People With Cancer and the People
Who Care About Them"
"Taking Part in Clinical Trials: What Cancer Patients Need to
Know"

Available in Spanish:
"Datos sobre el tratamiento de quimioterapia contra el cancer"
"El tratamiento de radioterapia; guia para el paciente durante el
tratamiento"
"En que consisten los estudios clinicos? Un folleto para los
pacientes de cancer"

The following pamphlets are available from the National
Comprehensive Cancer Network:
"Prostate Cancer Treatment Guidelines for Patients"
"Cancer Pain Treatment Guidelines for Patients"
"Nausea and Vomiting Treatment Guidelines for Patient
with Cancer"

Available in Spanish:
"Cáncer de la próstata"
"El dolor asociado con el cáncer"

Erectile Dysfunction Books and Pamphlets

"The Treatment of Organic Erectile Dysfunction: A Patient's
Guide." The American Urological Association Erectile Dys-
function Clinical Guidelines Panel. Copies can be obtained
from the AUA Health Policy Department at the address listed
in the beginning of appendix.
Levine SB. *Sexuality in Mid-Life*. New York: Plenum Press,
1998.
Levine SB. *Sexual Life: A Clnician's Guide (Critical Issues in
Psychiatry)*. New York: Plenum Press, 1992.
Rosen RC, Leiblum SR, eds. *Erectile Disorders: Assessment and
Treatment*. New York: Guildford Press, 1992.

Glossary

A

Abarelix: A GnRH antagonist under investigation as a hormone therapy for prostate cancer.

Abdomen: The part of the body below the ribs and above the pelvic bone that contains organs such as the intestines, the liver, the kidneys, the stomach, the bladder, and the prostate.

Active surveillance: An alternative to immediate treatment for men with presumed low-risk prostate cancer. Involves close monitoring and withholding active treatment unless there is a significant change in the patient's symptoms or PSA.

Acute urinary retention: The inability to pass urine from the bladder.

Acquired anorgasmia: A secondary inability to have an orgasm i.e., secondary to the side effects of medical therapy.

Adenocarcinoma: A form of cancer that develops from a malignant abnormality in the cells lining a glandular organ such as the prostate; almost all prostate cancers are adenocarcinomas.

Adrenal glands: Glands located above each kidney. These glands produce several different hormones including sex hormones.

Alendronate (Zoladex): An LHRH medication that comes in a pellet form, which is placed just under the skin. It is used to lower testosterone levels in men with advanced prostate cancer.

Alfuzosin (uroxatral): An alpha-blocker used to treat BPH.

Alkaline phosphatase: Chemical (**enzyme**) that is produced in the liver and bones. It is often elevated when prostate cancer has spread to the bones.

Alpha-blockers: A group of medications that may be used to treat the symptoms of benign prostate enlargement. They include doxazosin (Cardura), terazosin (Hytrin), silodosin (Rapaflo), and tamsulosin (Flowmax).

Alpha receptors: Regions/molecules on the bladder and prostate that when certain chemicals bind to mediate bladder and prostate function and tone.

Alprostadil: Prostaglandin E_1. For the treatment of erectile dysfunction, alprostadil comes in several forms—specifically, a suppository that is placed into the urethra (MUSE) or a liquid form that is delivered by intracavernous injection (Caverject or Edex).

Androderm: A topical form (patch) of testosterone used for testosterone replacement therapy.

Androgel: A gel form of testosterone replacement therapy.

Androgen blockade: Therapy to prevent the effects of the male hormones (androgens).

Androgens: Hormones that are necessary for the development and function of the male sexual organs and male sexual characteristics (i.e., hair, voice change).

Anejaculation: An inability to ejaculate.

Anesthesia: The loss of feeling or sensation. With respect to surgery, means the loss of sensation of pain, as it is induced to allow surgery or other painful procedures to be performed. *General*: A state of unconsciousness, produced by anesthetic agents, with absence of pain sensation over the entire body and a greater or lesser degree of muscle relaxation. *Local*: Anesthesia confined to one part of the body. *Spinal*: Anesthesia produced by injection of a local anesthetic into the subarachnoid space around the spinal cord.

Aneurysm: Pertaining to a penile prosthesis, an abnormal dilation of the prosthesis related to weakening of a part of the cylinder.

Angina: Pain in the chest, with a feeling of suffocation, that occurs with decreased blood flow and oxygenation to the heart.

Anorexia: Loss of appetite.

Anorgasmia: Failure to experience an orgasm during sex. *See also* acquired anorgasmia and congenital anorgasmia.

Antiandrogen: Drugs that counteract the action of testosterone.

Antidepressant: Medication prescribed to relieve depression.

Antigen: A substance that stimulates the individual's body to produce cells that fight off the antigen, and in doing so, kill cancer cells.

Antioxidant: A chemical that helps prevent changes in cells and reduce damage to the cell that can cause it to become cancerous.

Anus: The outside opening of the rectum.

Apex of the prostate: The end of the prostate gland located farthest away from the urinary bladder.

Arteriography: A test for identifying and locating arterial disease in the penis, using injected contrast to find constricted or blocked arteries.

Artery: A blood vessel that carries oxygenated blood from the heart to other parts of the body.

Artificial urinary sphincter: A prosthesis designed to restore continence in an incontinent person by constricting the urethra.

Atherosclerosis: Hardening of the arteries, often related to smoking and elevated cholesterol.

Autoinflation: Pertaining to a penile prosthesis, the spontaneous inflation of the prosthesis without manual pumping.

Axial rigidity: The rigidity as measured along the axis or length of the penis.

B

Benign: A growth that is not cancerous.

Benign prostatic hyperplasia: *See* BPH.

Bicalutamide: The generic name for Casodex, an antiandrogen.

BID: Twice a day.

Bilateral: Both sides.

Biochemical progression: Recurrence of prostate cancer as defined by an elevation in PSA.

Biopsy: The removal of small sample(s) of tissue for examination under the microscope.

Biphosphonate: A type of medication that is used to treat osteoporosis and the bone pain caused by some types of cancer.

Bladder: The hollow organ that stores and discharges urine from the body.

Bladder catheterization: Passage of a catheter into the urinary bladder to drain urine.

Bladder compliance: The ability of the bladder to hold increasing amounts of urine without increases in bladder pressure; reflects the elasticity of the bladder.

Bladder neck: The outlet area of the bladder. It is comprised of circular muscle fibers and helps in the control of urine.

Bladder neck contracture: Scar tissue at the bladder neck that causes narrowing.

Bladder outlet: The first part of the natural channel through which urine passes when it leaves the bladder.

Bladder outlet obstruction: Obstruction of the bladder outlet causing problems with urination and/or retention of urine in the bladder.

Bladder spasm: A sudden contraction of the bladder, which one is not able to control, that often produces pain and a feeling of the need to urinate.

Bladder stones: Stones present in the bladder.

Bladder ultrasound: A test done using an ultrasound to see how much urine is left in the bladder after voiding, the postvoid residual.

Bone scan: A specialized nuclear medicine study that allows one to detect changes in the bone that may be related to metastatic prostate cancer.

Bound PSA: PSA attached to the proteins in the bloodstream.

Bowel prep: Cleansing (and sterilization) of the intestines before abdominal surgery.

BPH (benign prostatic hyperplasia): Noncancerous enlargement of the prostate.

Brachytherapy: A form of radiation therapy whereby radioactive pellets are placed into the prostate.

Butterfly needle: A small needle that has tubing attached to it.

C

Cancer: Abnormal and uncontrolled growth of cells in the body that may spread, injure areas of the body, and lead to death.

Capsule: A fibrous outer layer that surrounds the prostate.

Carcinoma: A form of cancer that originates from epithelial tissues, such as colon, skin, lungs, prostate, bladder; *see* adenocarcinoma.

Casodex: The brand name for bicalutamide, an antiandrogen.

Castration: The surgical removal of both testicles.

Catheter: A hollow tube that allows for fluid drainage from or injection into an area.

Catheterization: The passage of a catheter into the bladder to empty the bladder of urine.

Caverject: A form of injection therapy produced by Pfizer. It contains prostaglandin E_1.

Cavernosography: A technique used to visualize areas of venous leak. It involves the injection of a cavernous smooth-muscle dilator (e.g., prostaglandin E_1 or trimix), followed by placement of a butterfly needle into the corpora, instillation of a contrast agent into the corpora, and x-ray photographs to visualize the sites of venous leak.

Cavernosometry: A somewhat invasive technique used to determine whether a venous leak is present.

Cell: The smallest unit of the body. Tissues in the body are made up of cells.

Central nervous system: The portion of the nervous system consisting of the brain and the spinal cord.

cGMP: A neurotransmitter that causes relaxation of the arteries and smooth muscles in the penis to permit increased blood flow into the penis.

Chemoprevention: The use of a substance to prevent the development and growth of cancer.

Chemotherapy: A treatment for cancer that uses powerful medications to weaken and destroy the cancer cells.

Cholesterol: A fat-like substance that is important to certain body functions but that, when present in excessive amounts, contributes to unhealthy fatty deposits in the arteries that may interfere with blood flow.

Chromosome: Part of the cell that carries genes and functions in the transmission of hereditary information.

Cialis: *See* tadalafil.

Clean intermittent catheterization (CIC): The placement of a catheter into the bladder to drain urine and the removal after the urine is drained at defined intervals throughout the day, to allow for bladder emptying. It may also be performed to maintain patency after treatment of a bladder neck contracture or urethral stricture.

Clinical trials: A carefully planned experiment to evaluate a treatment or medication (often a new drug) for an unproven use.

Colostomy: A surgical opening between the colon (large intestine) and the skin that allows stool to drain into a collecting bag.

Complication: An undesirable result of a treatment, surgery, or medication.

Conformal EBRT: EBRT that uses CT scan images to better visualize radiation targets and normal tissues.

Congenital anorgasmia: A rare form of anorgasmia that is thought to be a product of an overly strict or repressive attitude toward sex.

Congestive heart failure: An inability of the heart to pump blood adequately, leading to swelling and fluid in the lungs.

Contracture: Scarring which can occur at the bladder neck after radical prostatectomy or radiation therapy and result in decreased force of urine stream and incomplete bladder emptying.

Corona: The area of the penis just before the glans.

Corpora cavernosa: The two cylindrical structures in the penis that are composed of the penile erectile tissue. They are located on the top of the penis (singular: corpus cavernosum).

Corpus spongiosum: One of the three cylindrical structures in the penis. The urethra passes through the corpus spongiosum. It is not involved in erections.

Cryotherapy, cryosurgery: A prostate cancer therapy in which the prostate is frozen to destroy the cancer cells.

CT scan/CAT scan (computerized tomography/computerized axial tomography): A specialized x-ray study that allows one to visualize internal structures in cross-section to look for abnormalities.

Cystoscope: A telescope-like instrument that allows one to examine the urethra and inside of the bladder.

Cystoscopy: The procedure of using a cystoscope to look into the urethra and bladder.

D

Degarelix (Firmagon): a new LHRH analog hormonal therapy.

Debulk: To decrease the amount of cancer present by surgery, hormone therapy, or chemotherapy.

Deep venous thrombosis (DVT): The formation of a blood clot in the large deep veins, usually of the legs or in the pelvis.

Deferred therapy: Delaying treatment until the cancer appears to be a threat to the patient.

Delayed ejaculation: Taking a longer time to ejaculate. This effect is seen with some antidepressants.

Depression: A mental state of depressed mood characterized by feelings of sadness, despair, and discouragement.

Detumescence: Subsidence of swelling or turgor; with respect to erections, loss of rigidity.

Diabetes mellitus: A chronic disease associated with high levels of sugar (glucose) in the blood.

Diagnosis: The identification of the cause or presence of a medical problem or disease.

Diethylstilbestrol (DES): A form of the female hormone estrogen.

Digital rectal examination (DRE): The examination of the prostate by placing a gloved finger into the rectum.

Dihydrotestosterone (DHT): A breakdown product of testosterone, which stimulates the prostate to grow.

Disease: Any change from or interruption of the normal structure or function of any part, organ, or system of the body that presents with characteristic symptoms and signs, and whose cause and prognosis may be known or unknown.

Dissection: The surgical removal of tissue.

Docetaxel: A type of chemotherapy, a taxane, that has been shown to be effective in hormone refractory prostate cancer.

Doppler ultrasonography: Use of a Doppler probe during ultrasound to look at flow through vessels.

Double-blind: Pertaining to a study, a situation in which neither the patient nor the physician is aware of which medication the patient is receiving.

Doubling time: The amount of time that it takes for the cancer to double in size.

Down-size: To shrink or reduce the size of the cancer.

Down-stage: To reduce the initial stage of the cancer to a lower (better prognostic) stage.

Doxazosin (Cardura): An alpha-blocker used to treat BPH.

Dutasteride (Avodart): A 5-alpha-reductase inhibitor used to treat BPH. It has been shown to decrease the risk of prostate cancer.

E

EBRT: *See* external beam radiation therapy.

Edex: Alprostadil alfadex. A form of injection therapy produced by Schwarz Pharma. It contains prostaglandin E_1 and works via the same mechanism as Caverject.

Efficacy: The power or ability to produce an effect.

Ejaculation: The release of semen through the penis during orgasm. After radical prostatectomy and often after a TURP, no fluid is released during orgasm.

Ejaculatory duct: The structure through which the ejaculate passes into the urethra.

Ejaculatory dysfunction: An abnormality of ejaculatory function, such as retrograde ejaculation, premature ejaculation, delayed ejaculation, or anejaculation.

Electroejaculation: Use of an electrical stimulus to induce ejaculation.

Electrovaporization: A procedure in which electric current is used to destroy prostate tissue.

Embolization: The introduction of a substance into a blood vessel in an attempt to obstruct (occlude) it.

Emission: A discharge, either voluntary or involuntary, of semen from the ejaculatory duct into the urethra.

Endorectal MRI: MRI study of the prostate that involves placing a probe into the rectum to better assess the prostate gland.

Enzyme: A chemical that is produced by living cells that causes chemical reactions to occur while not being changed itself.

Epidural anesthesia: A special type of anesthesia whereby pain medications are placed through a catheter in the back, into the fluid that surrounds the spinal cord.

Erectile dysfunction: The inability to achieve and/or maintain an erection satisfactory for the completion of sexual performance.

Erection: The process whereby the penis becomes rigid.

Erosion: Destruction of a tissue surface—for example, a penile prosthesis eroding through the skin.

Estramustine: An anticancer drug that stops growth of cells and eventually destroys them.

Estrogen: A female hormone.

Eulexin: The brand name for flutamide, an antiandrogen.

Experimental: An untested or unproven treatment or approach to treatment.

External-beam radiation therapy (EBRT): Use of radiation that passes through the skin and is focused for maximal effect on a target organ, such as the prostate, to kill cancer cells.

Extravasation: A discharge or escape of fluid, normally found in a vessel or tube, into the surrounding tissue.

F

FDA: Food and Drug Administration. Agency responsible for the approval of prescription medications in the United States.

Firmagon: *See* Degarelix.

Fistula: An abnormal passage or communication, usually between two internal organs, or leading from an internal organ to the surface of the body.

Flare reaction: A temporary increase in tumor growth and symptoms that is caused by the initial use of LHRH agonists. It is prevented by the use of an antiandrogen 1 week before LHRH agonist therapy begins.

Fluoroscopy: Use of a fluoroscope, a radiologic device that is used for examining deep structures by means of x-rays.

Flutamide (Eulexin): An antiandrogen that is taken three times a day to provide total androgen blockade, blocking the effects of androgens made by the adrenals.

Foley catheter: A latex or silicone catheter that drains urine from the bladder.

Free PSA: The PSA present that is not bound to proteins. It is often expressed as a ratio of free PSA to total PSA in terms of percent, which is the free PSA divided by the total PSA × 100.

Frequency: A term used to describe the need to urinate eight or more times per day.

Frozen section: A preliminary quick evaluation of tissue, removed at the time of biopsy or during surgery, by the pathologist who freezes the sample of tissue and shaves off a thin slice to examine under the microscope.

G

GAQ: *See* global assessment questionnaire.

Gastrointestinal (GI): Related to the digestive system and/or the intestines.

Gender: The category to which an individual is assigned on the basis of sex, either male or female.

Gene therapy: The deliberate alteration of genes in an attempt to affect their function.

General anesthesia: Anesthesia which involves total loss of consciousness.

Genetics: A field of medicine that studies heredity.

Genitalia, male: The external sexual organs—in the male, the penis, testes, epididymis, and vas deferens.

Genitourinary tract: The urinary system (kidney, ureters and bladder, and urethra) and the genitalia (in the male the prostate, seminal vesicles, vas deferens, and testicles).

Gland: A structure or organ that produces substances that affect other areas of the body.

Glans: The tip of the penis.

Gleason grade: A commonly used method to classify how cells appear in cancerous prostate tissues; the less the cancerous cells look like normal cells, the more malignant the cancer; two numbers, each from 1 to 5, are assigned to the two most predominant types of cells present. These two numbers are added together to produce the **Gleason score**. Higher numbers indicate more aggressive cancers.

Global assessment questionnaire (GAQ): A self-administered questionnaire that allows patients to rate improvement in erectile function.

Glycosylated end-products: A chemical associated with diabetes that may contribute to erectile dysfunction by decreasing nitric oxide activity.

Glycosylated hemoglobin: A chemical in the blood that allows monitoring of blood sugar control in individuals with diabetes mellitus. An elevated $HgbA_{1c}$ is indicative of poor blood sugar control.

GnRH (LHRH) antagonist: A form of hormone therapy which works at the level of the brain to directly suppress the production of testosterone without initially raising the testosterone level.

Goserelin acetate (Zoladex): An LHRH analogue used in the treatment of advanced prostate cancer.

Groin: The area between the lower abdomen and the thigh.

Gynecomastia: Enlargement or tenderness of the male breast(s).

H

Hardening of the arteries: Descriptive expression that commonly refers to a group of diseases (forms of arteriosclerosis) characterized by abnormal thickening and hardening (sclerosis) of arterial walls, in which the arteries lose their elasticity. If the thickening/hardening is significant, it may interfere with blood flow.

Hematoma: A blister-like collection of blood under the skin.

Hematospermia: The presence of blood in the ejaculate (semen).

Hematuria: The presence of blood in the urine. It may be gross (visible) or microscopic (only detected under the microscope).

Hemibody: Half of the body.

Hereditary: Inherited from one's parents or earlier generations.

Heredity: The passage of characteristics from parents to their children by genes (genetic material).

Hernia: A weakening in the muscle that leads to a bulge, often in the groin.

Hesitancy: A delay in the start of the urine stream during voiding.

High-density lipoprotein (HDL): "Good" cholesterol.

High-flow priapism: Priapism that occurs secondary to increased arterial flow.

High grade: Very advanced cancer cells.

High intensity focused ultrasonography: A form of prostate cancer therapy that involves focusing high intensity ultrasound into the prostate to heat the prostate and destroy prostate cancer cells. It is being used in Europe but has not been approved in the United States.

High risk: More likely to have a complication or side effect.

History: An oral or written interview that consists of questions about your medical, social, and sexual background.

Histrelin acetate (Vantas): A type of LHRH analogue used for treatment of advanced prostate cancer.

Hormone refractory: Prostate cancer that is resistant to hormone therapy.

Hormone resistant: Prostate cancer that is resistant to hormone therapy.

Hormone therapy: The manipulation of the disease's natural history and symptoms by altering hormone levels.

Hormones: Substances (estrogens and androgens) responsible for secondary sex characteristics (hair growth and voice change in men).

Hot flashes: The sudden feeling of being warm, may be associated with sweating and flushing of the skin, which occurs with hormone therapy.

Hydronephrosis: Dilation of the kidneys, usually due to obstruction.

Hypercholesterolemia: An excess of cholesterol in the blood.

Hyperplasia: Enlargement of an organ or tissue because of an increase in the number of cells in that organ or tissue; an example is benign prostatic hyperplasia.

Hyperprolactinemia: A condition characterized by excess prolactin production. It may be related to a tumor of the pituitary gland but also may be caused by certain medications.

Hypertension: High blood pressure.

Hyperthermia: Heating of the prostate to destroy tissue.

Hypoechoic: In ultrasonography, giving off few echoes; said of tissues or structures that reflect relatively few ultrasound waves directed at them.

Hypogonadism: A condition in which the testes are not producing adequate testosterone. It may occur because of a testicular problem or because of a lack of stimulation of the testes by the brain.

Hyponatremic: A low sodium level in the blood.

Hypotension: Low blood pressure: May be associated with dizziness, fast heart rate and feeling weak and faint.

I

Iatrogenic: Resulting from treatment by a physician, such as from medications, procedures, or surgery.

ICU (intensive care unit): A specialized area of the hospital where critically ill patients are taken care of.

IM: Intramuscular.

Immune system: A complex group of organs, tissues, blood cells and substances that work to fight off infections, cancers or foreign substances.

Impotence: *See* erectile dysfunction.

Incidence: The rate at which a certain event occurs—for example, the number of new cases of a specific disease that occur during a certain period.

Incidental: Insignificant or irrelevant.

Incision: Cutting of the skin at the beginning of surgery.

Incontinence: Leakage of a substance without control. If the substance is urine, it is called urinary incontinence; if stool, it's called fecal incontinence. There are various kinds and degrees of urinary incontinence:

• *Overflow incontinence* is a condition in which the bladder retains urine after voiding, and as a result, urine leaks out, similar to a full cup under the faucet.

• *Stress incontinence* is the involuntary leakage of urine during periods of increased bladder pressure, such as coughing, laughing, and sneezing.

Indications: The reasons for undertaking a specific treatment.

Infarct: An area of dead tissue resulting from a sudden loss of its blood supply.

Inflammation: Swelling, redness, pain, and irritation as the result of injury, infection, or surgery.

Informed consent: Permission given by a patient for a particular treatment after the patient has been notified of the indications for the procedure, the possible benefits and risks of the procedure, and alternative procedures that could be performed for the patient's condition.

Inpatient: A patient who is admitted to the hospital for treatment.

Insulin-dependent diabetes mellitus: Diabetes in which the body does not produce sufficient insulin.

Integrative treatment: Treatments that are designed to work together.

Intermittency: An inability to complete voiding and emptying the bladder with one single contraction of the bladder. A stopping and starting of the urine stream during urination.

Internist: A medical doctor who specializes in the nonsurgical treatment of disease and disease prevention.

Interposition: The act of placing between.

Interstitial: Within an organ, such as interstitial brachytherapy, whereby radioactive seeds are placed into the prostate.

Intracavernous: Into the corpora cavernosa.

Intracavernous pressure: The pressure within the corpora cavernosa, as measured during cavernosography.

Intramuscular (IM): Pertaining to the muscles; injection into the muscle.

Intraurethral: Placed into the urethra.

Intraurethral alprostadil: *See* MUSE.

Intravenous: Into the veins.

Invasive: In cancer, means the spread of the cancer beyond the site where it initially developed into surrounding tissues.

Investigational: *See* experimental.

Investigator: A doctor or other individual who is involved with an experimental study or clinical trial.

Ischemia: A deficiency of blood flow to an area that compromises the health of the tissue.

IV: Intravenous.

IVP (intravenous pyelogram): A radiologic study, in which a contrast material (dye) is injected into the veins and is picked up by the kidneys and passed out into the urine, which allows one to visualize the urinary tract.

K

Kegel exercises (pelvic floor muscle exercises): Exercises that help one strengthen muscles that aid in the control of urinary incontinence.

Kidney: One of a pair of organs responsible for eliminating chemicals and fluid from the body.

L

Laparoscopic radical prostatectomy: Removal of the entire prostate, seminal vesicles, and part of the vas deferens via the laparoscope.

Laparoscopic: Performed with a laparoscope.

Laparoscopy: Surgery performed through small incisions with visualization provided by a small fiberoptic instrument and fine instruments that fit through the small incisions.

Laser: A concentrated beam of high-energy light that is used in surgery.

Leukemia: A cancer of the blood-forming organs that affects the blood cells.

Leuprolide: An LHRH analogue that is administered once every 28, 84, 112 days, or yearly to lower testosterone levels for the treatment of advanced prostate cancer.

Levitra: *See* vardenafil.

LH: *See* luteinizing hormone.

LHRH analogue: A medication that tells the brain to tell the testicles to stop producing testosterone. It may initially raise serum testosterone, thus it is combined initially with an antiandrogen in men with metastatic prostate cancer.

LHRH antagonist: *See* GnRH antagonist.

Libido: Sex drive, interest in sex.

Lifestyle: The way a person chooses to live.

Lobe: A part of an organ. There are five distinct lobes in the prostate: two lateral lobes, one middle, an anterior, and a posterior.

Local anesthesia: Control of pain in a localized area of the body.

Local recurrence: The return of cancer to the area where it was first identified.

Localized: Confined, limited, contained to a specific area.

Lower urinary tract symptoms (LUTS): Symptoms that may be storage (urgency, frequency, urgency incontinence, nocturia) or voiding (hesitancy, intermittency, weak stream, postvoid dribbling, straining to void) symptoms.

Low-flow priapism: Priapism that occurs secondary to venous outflow obstruction.

Low-grade: Cancer that does not appear aggressive, advanced.

Luteinizing hormone (LH): A chemical produced by the brain that stimulates the testes to produce testosterone.

Lycopene: A substance found in tomatoes that has anticancer effects on the prostate.

Lymph: A clear fluid that is found throughout the body. Lymph fluid helps fight infections.

Lymph node(s): Small bean-shaped glands that are found throughout the body. Lymph fluid passes through the lymph nodes, which filter out bacteria, cancer cells, and toxic chemicals.

Lymph node dissection: In the case of prostate cancer, pelvic lymph node dissection, which is the surgical removal of the lymph nodes in the pelvis to determine if prostate cancer has spread to the these nodes.

Lymphadenectomy: The technical term for lymph node dissection.

Lymphangiography: An x-ray test in which contrast is injected into the lymph vessels to determine if there is any blockage/tumor spread to the lymph nodes.

Lymphocele: A collection of lymph fluid in an area of the body.

M

Malignancy: Cancer. Uncontrolled growth of cells that can spread to other areas of the body and cause death.

Malignant: Cancerous, with the potential for uncontrolled growth and spread.

Medical oncologist: *See* oncologist.

Megace (megestrol): A medication that is used to treat hot flashes associated with hormone therapy.

Metastatic cancer: Cancer that has spread outside of the organ or structure in which it arose to another area of the body.

Metastatic recurrence: The return of cancer in an area of the body that is not the site where it originally developed.

Metastases: *See* metastatic cancer.

Microscopic: Small enough that a microscope is needed to see it.

Migration: Spontaneous change of place.

Mitoxantrone: An anticancer drug that belongs to a family of drugs called antitumor antibiotics. It interferes with the growth of cancer cells.

Moderately differentiated: An intermediate grade of cancer as based on pathological evaluation of the tissue.

Molecular biology: The part of biology that deals with the formation, structure, and activity of macromolecules that are essential for life, such as nucleic acids.

Morbidity: Unhealthy results and complications resulting from treatment.

Mortality: Death related to disease or treatment.

MRI (magnetic resonance imaging): A study that is similar to a CT scan in that it allows one to see internal structures in detail, but it does not involve radiation.

Multifocal: Found in more than one area.

MUSE: Intraurethral alprostadil; a small suppository that comes preloaded in a small applicator that is placed into the tip of the penis. The small button at the other end of the suppository is squeezed to release the suppository into the urethra. Gentle rubbing of the penis causes the suppository to dissolve. The prostaglandin is then absorbed through the urethral mucosa and passes into the corpora cavernosa, where it stimulates blood flow into the penis through the cAMP pathway.

Myth: A popular belief or tradition that is unfounded and unproven.

N

NAION: *See* nonarteritic ischemic optic neuropathy.

Negative: A test result that does not show what one is looking for.

Neoadjuvant therapy: The use of a treatment, such as chemotherapy, hormone therapy, and radiation therapy, before surgery.

Neoplastic: Malignant, cancerous.

Nephrostomy tube: A tube that is placed through the back into the kidney and allows for drainage of urine from that kidney.

Neridronate (Nerixia): A type of biphosphonate. *See* biphosphonate.

Nerve: A cordlike structure composed of a collection of nerve fibers that conveys impulses between a part of the central nervous system and some other region of the body.

Nerve-sparing: With regard to prostate cancer, it is the attempt to not damage or remove the nerves that lie on either side of the prostate gland that are in part responsible for normal erections. Injury to the nerves can cause erectile dysfunction.

Nerve-sparing prostatectomy: Form of radical prostatectomy whereby an attempt is made to spare the nerves involved in erectile function.

Neurogenic bladder: A bladder that has an abnormality in its nerve supply.

Neurologic: Pertaining to the brain or nerves.

Neurotransmitter: A chemical released from a nerve cell that transmits an impulse to another nerve, cell, or organ.

Nilandron: The brand name for nilutamide, an antiandrogen.

Nitrate: A form of nitric acid that causes dilation (opening up) of the blood vessels to the heart. Nitroglycerin is a form of nitrate.

Nitric oxide: A chemical in the body that stimulates production of cGMP, which is necessary for erectile function.

Nitroglycerin: A medication that is usually taken sublingually (under the tongue) for the relief of angina. It may also be applied to the chest in a paste form for the prevention of angina.

Nocturia: Awakening one or more times at night with the desire to void.

Nocturnal: Occurring or active at night.

Nocturnal penile tumescence (NPT) study: A specialized study that evaluates the frequency and the quality of nocturnal erections.

Nonarteritic ischemic optic neuropathy (NAION): A sudden, painless loss of vision in one or both eyes. The cause is reduced blood flow to the optic nerve.

Noninsulin-dependent diabetes mellitus: Diabetes in which the body does not respond adequately to insulin.

Noninvasive: Not requiring any incision or the insertion of an instrument or substance into the body.

Norepinephrine: A neurotransmitter that regulates the sympathetic nervous system.

Nucleic acids: Any of a group of complex compounds found in all living cells. Nucleic acids in the form of DNA and RNA control the functions of cells and heredity.

Nutrition: The science or study that deals with food and nourishment, especially in humans.

O

Objective: Perceptible to the external senses; something the physician uses to quantify, measure, or identify.

Obturator nerve: A nerve located in the pelvis near the pelvic lymph nodes that controls movement of the leg.

Occlusion: Blockage of flow.

Occult: Not detectable on gross examination.

Occult cancer: Cancer that is not detectable through standard physical exams; symptom-free disease.

Oral: Taken by mouth.

Oncologist: A medical specialist who is trained to evaluate and treat cancer.

Orchiectomy: Removal of the testicle(s).

Organ: Tissues in the body that work together to perform a specific function, e.g., the kidneys, bladder, heart.

Organ-confined disease: Prostate cancer that is apparently confined to the prostate clinically or pathologically; not going beyond the edges of the prostate capsule.

Orgasm: Sexual climax; the culmination of sexual excitement.

Orgasmic dysfunction: Alterations in orgasmic function or the inability to achieve an orgasm.

Orthostatic hypotension: The acute lowering of blood pressure when a person changes from a sitting or lying position to an upright position (standing). Also called postural hypotension.

Osteoblastic lesion: Pertaining to plain x-ray of a bone, increased density of bone seen on x-ray when there is extensive new bone formation due to cancerous destruction of the bone.

Osteolytic lesion: Pertaining to plain x-ray of a bone, refers to decreased density of bone seen on x-ray when there is destruction and loss of bone by cancer.

Osteoporosis: The reduction in the amount of bone mass, leading to fractures after minimal trauma.

Overactive bladder: A syndrome consisting of urgency with or without urgency incontinence; often with frequency and nocturia without an identifiable cause.

Overflow incontinence: A condition in which the bladder retains urine after voiding, and as a result, urine leaks out, similar to a full cup under the faucet.

P

Palliative: Treatment designed to relieve a particular problem without necessarily solving it, e.g., palliative therapy is given. in order to relieve symptoms and improve quality of life, but it does not cure the patient.

Palpable: Capable of being felt during a physical examination by an experienced doctor. In the case of prostate cancer, this refers to an abnormality of the prostate that can be felt during a rectal examination.

Palpation: Feeling with the hand or fingers, by applying light pressure.

PAP (prostatic acid phosphatase): A chemical that was once used to try to determine if the prostate cancer had spread outside of the prostate.

Parenteral: Administered not by mouth but rather by injection by some other route (e.g., intramuscular, subcutaneous).

Partin tables: Tables that are developed based on results of the PSA, clinical stage, and Gleason score involving thousands of men with prostate cancer. These tables are used to predict the likelihood that prostate cancer has spread to the lymph nodes or seminal vesicles, penetrated the capsule, or remains confined to the prostate. The tables were developed by Dr. Partin at Johns Hopkins University.

Pathologist: A doctor trained in the evaluation of tissues under the microscope to determine the presence/absence of disease.

PC SPES: An herbal therapy for prostate cancer that is comprised of eight different herbs.

PDE-5 inhibitor: *See* Phosphodiesterase type 5 inhibitor.

Pelvic floor muscle exercise: *See* Kegel exercises.

Pelvic lymph node dissection: A procedure to remove lymph nodes that prostate cancer typically spreads to.

Pelvis: The part of the body that is framed by the hip bones.

Penile arterial bypass surgery: A surgical procedure that provides an alternative pathway to bring blood flow into the penis and avoids the obstructed artery.

Penile prosthesis: A device that is surgically placed into the penis that allows a man with erectile dysfunction to have an erection.

Penis: The male organ that is used for urination and intercourse.

Percutaneous: Through the skin.

Perineal: Refers to an incision made behind the scrotum and in front of the anus: The prostate can be removed through a perineal incision.

Perineal prostatectomy: Removal of the entire prostate, seminal vesicles, and part of the vas deferens through an incision made in the perineum.

Perineum: The area of the body that is behind the scrotum and in front of the anus.

Periprostatic: That tissue that lies immediately adjacent to the prostate.

Permanent section: The formal preparation of tissue removed at the time of surgery for microscopic evaluation.

Peyronie's disease: A benign (non-cancerous) condition of the penis that tends to affect middle-aged men. It is characterized by the formation of plaques in the tunica albuginea of the penis and may cause erectile dysfunction.

Pharmacology: The science of drugs, including their composition, uses, and effects.

Phosphodiesterase type 5 (PDE-5): An enzyme that is responsible for the breakdown of cGMP. Inhibition of PDE-5 leads to a buildup of cGMP.

Phosphodiesterase type 5 (PDE-5) inhibitor: A chemical that prevents the function of PDE-5. The use of such an inhibitor leads to an increase in cGMP.

Physiologic: Functioning in a normal range for human physiology.

PIN (prostatic intraepithelial neoplasia): An abnormal area in a prostate biopsy specimen that is not cancerous, but may become cancerous or be associated with cancer elsewhere in the prostate.

Pituitary adenoma: A benign tumor of the pituitary gland. An adenoma of the anterior pituitary may produce excessive amounts of prolactin.

Pituitary gland: A gland in the brain that is composed of two parts (lobes), the anterior gland and the posterior gland. The anterior pituitary gland produces a variety of hormones, including luteinizing hormone and prolactin.

Placebo: A fake medication ("candy pill") or treatment that has no effect on the body that is often used in experimental studies to determine if the experimental medication/treatment has an effect.

Ploidy status: The genetic status of cells, similar to the grade.

Pneumatic sequential stockings: Inflatable stockings that squeeze the legs intermittently to decrease the risk of a blood clot in the legs.

Polycythemia: An increase in the total red blood cell mass in the blood.

Poorly differentiated: High-grade, aggressive cancer as determined by microscopic evaluation of the tissue.

Positive biopsy: For cancer, it is the detection of cancer in the tissue.

Positive margin: The presence of cancer cells at the cut edge of tissue removed during surgery. A positive margin indicates that there may be cancer cells remaining in the body.

Posterior: The rear or back side.

Postural hypotension: *See* orthostatic hypotension.

Premature ejaculation: Quick ejaculation. The fourth edition of the *American Psychiatric Association's Diagnostic and Statistical Manual* outlines three criteria for premature ejaculation: (1) persistent or repeated ejaculation occurs with slight stimulation before, on, or shortly after penetration and before the person wishes it; (2) the disturbance causes considerable anguish or interpersonal difficulty; and (3) the premature ejaculation is not due exclusively to the direct effects of a chemical.

Pressure/flow study: A component of a urodynamic study, whereby the bladder pressure is plotted against the urine flow rate. It is useful in determining if obstruction to the outflow of urine is present.

Prevalence: The number of cases of a disease that are present in a population at one given point in time.

Priapism: An erection that lasts longer than 4 to 6 hours.

Proctitis: Inflammation of the rectum.

Prognosis: The long-term outlook or prospect for survival and recovery from a disease.

Progression: The continued growth of cancer or disease.

Prolactin: One of the hormones produced by the pituitary gland. In males, elevated prolactin levels can lower testosterone levels, decrease libido, and affect erectile function.

Prolonged erection: An erection that lasts longer than 4 hours but less than 6 hours. It may be associated with the use of pharmacologic therapy for erectile dysfunction.

Proscar (finasteride): A drug that decreases prostate size. It is FDA approved for BPH; it has been shown to decrease the incidence of prostate cancer.

Prostaglandin E$_1$: A type of prostaglandin that increases the cAMP level, which causes smooth-muscle relaxation.

Prostate: A gland that surrounds the urethra and is located just under the bladder. It produces fluid that is part of the ejaculate (semen). This fluid provides some nutrient to the sperm.

Prostate specific antigen (PSA): A chemical produced by benign and cancerous prostate tissue. The level tends to be higher with prostate cancer.

Prostate surgery: Surgery for benign and malignant diseases of the prostate.

Prostatectomy: Any of several surgical procedures in which part or all of the prostate gland is removed. These procedures include laparoscopic radical prostatectomy, radical perineal prostatectomy, radical retropubic prostatectomy, and transurethral prostatectomy (TURP), and open prostatectomy for BPH either retropubic prostatectomy or suprapubic prostatectomy.

ProstaScint: A specialized study that detects an antigen called the prostate-specific antigen. It may be picking up recurrent prostate cancer.

Prostatic stents: Cylindrical devices that can be placed in the urethra to relieve prostatic obstruction.

Prostatitis: Inflammation or infection of the prostate gland.

Prosthesis: An artificial device used to replace the lost normal function of a structure or organ in the body.

Protocol: Research study used to evaluate a specific medication or treatment.

Proton-beam therapy: In conjunction with external-beam therapy, use of powerful beams of photons that are focused onto the prostate.

PSA density: The amount of PSA per gram of prostate tissue (PSA/g of prostate tissue).

PSA nadir: The lowest value that the PSA reaches during a particular treatment.

PSA progression: Increase in PSA after treatment of prostate cancer.

PSA velocity: The rate of change of the PSA over a period of time (change in PSA/change in time).

Psychogenic: Stemming from the mind or psyche.

Q

QD: Daily

QID: Four times a day

QOD: Every other day

Quality of life: An evaluation of healthy status relative to the patient's age, expectations, and physical and mental capabilities.

R

Radial rigidity: Rigidity across the width or radius of the penis.

Radiation oncologist: A physician who treats cancer through the use of radiation therapy.

Radiation proctitis: Inflammation of the rectal lining as a result of radiation therapy.

Radiation therapy: Use of radioactive beams or implants to kill cancer cells.

Radical perineal prostatectomy: Removal of the entire prostate and seminal vesicles for prostate cancer through a perineal incision.

Radical prostatectomy: A surgical procedure to remove the entire prostate and the seminal vesicles and part of the vas deferens to treat prostate cancer. May be performed via retropubic, laparoscopic, perineal, and robotic approaches.

Radical retropubic prostatectomy: The surgical removal of the entire prostate plus the seminal vesicles and part of the vas deferens through an incision that extends down from the umbilicus (belly button).

Randomized: The process of assigning patients to different forms of treatment in a research study in a random manner.

Rapid eye movement (REM): A phase in the sleep cycle. Nocturnal erections occur during this phase of sleep.

Recurrence: The reappearance of disease. The recurrence may be clinical (a physical finding) or laboratory (e.g., a rise in the PSA).

Red blood cells: The cells in the blood that carry oxygen to the tissues.

Refractory: Resistant to therapy.

Regression: Reduction in the size of a single tumor or reduction in the number and/or size of several tumors.

Resectionist: The physician (urologist) who use the resectoscope during a turp.

Resectoscope: An instrument used to remove (resect) prostate, bladder, or urethral tissue through the urethra.

Resistance: Opposition to blood flow out of the penis.

Retention: Difficulty in emptying the bladder of urine; may be complete, in which one is unable to void, or partial, in which urine is left in the bladder after voiding.

Retrograde ejaculation: A condition whereby the ejaculate passes backward into the bladder instead of forward out the tip of the penis. This problem frequently occurs after transurethral prostatectomy.

Retropubic prostatectomy: An open surgical procedure to remove benign prostatic tissue, useful with very large prostates, does not remove the entire prostate; only a radical prostatectomy removes the entire prostate.

Risk: The chance or probability that a particular event will or will not happen.

Rhinitis: An inflammation of the nasal passages.

Robotic-assisted radical prostatectomy: A radical prostatectomy performed with the assistance of a robot.

S

Salvage: A procedure intended to "rescue" a patient after a failed prior therapy, e.g., a salvage radical prostatectomy after failed external-beam therapy.

Screening: Examination or testing of a group of individuals to separate those who are well from those who have an undiagnosed disease or defect or who are at high risk.

Scrotum: The pouch of skin that contains the testicles.

Selective serotonin reuptake inhibitor (SSRI): A type of medication that is used for depression and for premature ejaculation. Commonly used SSRIs include sertraline, paroxetine, and fluoxetine.

Semen: The thick whitish fluid, produced by glands of the male reproductive system, that carries the sperm (reproductive cells) through the penis during ejaculation.

Seminal vesicles: Glandular structures that are located above and behind the prostate: They produce fluid that is part of the ejaculate.

Sensitivity: The probability that a diagnostic test can correctly identify the presence of a particular disease.

Sex hormones: Substances (estrogens and androgens) responsible for secondary sex characteristics (e.g., hair growth and voice change in males).

Sexual dysfunction: An abnormality in the function of any component of the sexual response cycle.

Sexual response cycle: In male the cycle of interest, arousal, climax, ejaculation, and detumescence.

Sickle cell disease/sickle cell trait: A genetically inherited condition in which red blood cells take on an abnormal shape (sickle) in response to decreased oxygenation, dehydration, and acidosis. This abnormal shape makes it difficult for the red blood cells to pass through the blood vessels and leads to blockages of the vessels, causing pain and ischemia to tissues. In the penis, it may lead to priapism. African Americans are at increased risk for sickle cell disease/trait.

Side effect: A reaction to a medication or treatment.

Sign: Objective evidence of a disease, i.e., something that the doctor identifies.

Sildenafil (Viagra): The first oral therapy, phosphodiesterase type V inhibitor, for the treatment of erectile dysfunction.

Silodosin (Rapaflo): An alpha-blocker used to treat BPH.

Sinusoid: A blood-filled cavernous space. In the penis, these spaces are separated by a network of connective tissues containing muscle cells, small arteries, veins, and nerves.

Sleep apnea: A condition in which a person stops breathing for a short period of time during sleep (anywhere from a few seconds to a minute or two), causing him to wake repeatedly and get insufficient sleep.

Somnolence: Sleepiness, unnatural drowsiness.

Soy: Soy products are made from soy beans, a legume. Soy products are high in isoflavones, which may be helpful in preventing cancer cell growth.

Specificity: The probability that a diagnostic test can correctly identify the absence of disease.

Sperm: The cells in the male ejaculate that are produced by the testes that fertilize eggs.

Sphincter: A muscle that surrounds and by its tightening causes closure of an opening, e.g., the sphincter at the bladder outlet and in the urethra.

SSRI: *See* selective serotonin reuptake inhibitor.

Stage: A term used to describe the size and the extent of a cancer.

Staging: The process of determining the extent of disease, which is helpful in determining the most appropriate treatment. Often involves physical examination, blood testing, and x-ray studies.

Stress incontinence: The involuntary loss of urine during sudden rises in intra-abdominal pressure, e.g., with coughing, laughing, sneezing, or picking up heavy objects.

Striant: A transbuccal form of testosterone replacement therapy.

Stricture: Scarring as a result of a procedure or an injury that causes narrowing and in the case of the urethra may constrict the flow of urine.

Subjective: Pertaining to or perceived by the affected individual, but not perceptible to the other senses of another person.

Supplement: Something that completes or is an addition. A medication/therapy that is used in addition to another medication/therapy.

Supraphysiologic: Higher than the normal functional state or level in the body.

Suprapubic prostatectomy: An open surgical procedure for removing benign prostatic tissue, useful with very large prostates. Unlike a radical prostatectomy the entire prostate is not removed.

Suprapubic tube: A type of catheter placed percutaneously (through the skin) into the bladder through the lower abdominal wall in order to drain urine.

Suramin: An anticancer drug that may be helpful in metastatic cancer.

Symptom: Subjective evidence of a disease, i.e., something a patient describes, e.g., pain in abdomen.

Syncope: A temporary loss of consciousness.

T

Tadalafil (Cialis): An oral therapy, phosphodiesterase type V inhibitor, used for the treatment of erectile dysfunction. It has a longer half-life than the other oral therapies.

Tamsulosin (Flomax): An alpha-blocker used to treat BPH.

Taxane: A drug that inhibits cell growth by stopping cell division.

Terazosin (Hytrin): An alpha–blocker used to treat BPH.

Testim: A gel form of testosterone replacement therapy.

Testis: One of two male reproductive organs that are located within the scrotum and produce testosterone and sperm.

Testoderm: A topical form (patch) of testosterone used for testosterone replacement therapy.

Testosterone: The male hormone or androgen that is produced primarily by the testes and is needed for sexual function and fertility.

Three-dimensional (3-D) conformal radiation therapy: A variation of external-beam radiation therapy in which a computer, CT scan images, and a brace are used to focus the radiation more directly on the target organ/location.

TID: Three times a day.

Tissue: Specific type of material in the body, e.g., muscle, hair.

Total androgen blockade: The total blockage of all male hormones (those produced by the testicles and the adrenals) using surgery and/or medications.

Total PSA: The combination of bound and free PSA.

TNM system: Tumor, nodes, and metastases. The most common stagin system for prostate cancer.

Transdermal: Entering through the skin, as in administration of a drug applied to the skin in an ointment, gel, or patch form.

Transferrin: A chemical in the body that has been shown to stimulate the growth of prostate cancer.

Transperineal: Through the perineum.

Transrectal: Through the rectum.

Transrectal ultrasound: Visualization of the prostate by the use of an ultrasound probe placed into the rectum.

Transurethral: Through the urethra.

Transurethral incision of the prostate: A method of treating prostatic obstruction using an incision instead of resection; also known as TUIP.

Transurethral prostatectomy: *See* TURP.

Trazodone: A psychiatric medication that has been reported to cause priapism.

Triptorelin pamoate (Trelstar): An LHRH analogue used in the management of advanced prostate cancer.

Tumescence: Condition of being tumid or swollen; with respect to erections, penile rigidity.

Tumor: Abnormal tissue growth that may be cancerous or noncancerous (benign).

Tumor markers: Chemicals that can be used to detect and follow the treatment of certain cancers.

Tumor volume: The amount of cancer present in an organ.

Tunica albuginea: The dense, fibrous, elastic sheath enclosing the corpora cavernosa in the penis. Compression of small veins against the tunica albuginea during erection prevents the outflow of blood from the corpora, causing the penis to be rigid.

TURP (transurethral prostatectomy): A surgical technique performed under anesthesia using a specialized instrument similar to the cystoscope that allows the surgeon to remove the prostatic tissue that is bulging into the urethra and blocking the flow of urine through the urethra. After a TURP, the outer rim of the prostate remains.

U

Ultrasound: A technique used to look at internal organs by measuring reflected sound waves.

Undergrading: A term that indicates that the grade of cancer is worse than that found in the biopsy tissue.

Understaging: The assignment of an overly low clinical stage at initial diagnosis because of the difficulty of assessing the available information with accuracy.

Unit: Term referring to a pint of blood.

Ureters: Tubes that connect the kidneys to the bladder, through which urine passes into the bladder.

Urethra: The tube that runs from the bladder neck to the tip of the penis through which urine passes.

Urgency: A sudden compelling desire to urinate that is difficult to defer.

Urge Incontinence: associated with urgency.

Urinary incontinence: The loss of control of urine.

Urinary retention (acute): The inability to urinate leading to a filled bladder.

Urodynamics test: A test that assesses how well the bladder functions.

Uroflow: A measurement of the flow rate and volume of urine voided.

Urologist: A doctor that specializes in the evaluation and treatment of diseases of the genitourinary tract in men and women.

V

Vacuum device: A device that is used to provide an erection. It consists of three parts: a cylinder, a pump, and a constricting band.

Vardenafil (Levitra): An oral therapy, phosphodiesterase type V inhibitor, used in the management of erectile dysfunction.

Vascular: Pertaining to blood vessels.

Vas deferens: A pair of tiny tubes that connects each testicle to the urethra through which sperm passes.

Vasectomy: A procedure in which the vas deferens are cut and tied off, clipped, or cauterized to prevent the exit of sperm from the testicles. It makes a man sterile.

Vasoactive: Affecting the size (diameter) of blood vessels.

Vasospasm: Constriction of the arteries.

Vasovagal attack: A transient vascular and neurogenic reaction marked by pallor (white, ghost-like look), sweating, slow heart rate, and lowering of the blood pressure.

Vein: A blood vessel in the body that carries deoxygenated blood from the tissues back to the heart.

Venlafaxine: An antidepressant that is helpful in managing hot flashes associated with hormone therapy.

Venous leak: The situation in which veins do not compress to prevent blood from draining out of the corpora during erection. Venous leak may also refer to the rare occasions in which abnormally located veins allow for persistent drainage of blood during an erection.

Venous ligation surgery: A surgical procedure in which leaky veins in the penis are ligated to prevent blood from continually flowing out of the penis during erection.

Viadur: An LHRH analogue that is administered by implant yearly to lower testosterone levels for the treatment of advanced prostate cancer.

Viagra: *See* sildenafil.

W

Wasting: An indentation in the penis.

Watchful waiting: Active observation and regular monitoring of a patient without actual treatment.

Well-differentiated: A low-grade.

X

X-ray: A type of high-energy radiation that can be used at low levels to make images of the internal structure of the body and at high levels for radiation therapy.

Z

Zoladex: *See* goserelin acetate.

Zoledronate (zometa): A biphosphonate that increases bone density in men on hormonal therapy.

Index

benzodiazepines, as cause of ED, 180
bicalutamide (Casodex), 98, 100–101
biochemical recurrence, after treatment of
    prostate cancer, 113, 114
biopsy. *See* TRUS (transurethral
    ultrasound)-guided biopsy
bisphosphonates
    for bone pain, 120
    for osteoporosis prevention, 104–105
bladder
    cystoscopy of, 126–127
    hypertrophy of, 131
bladder compliance, cystometrogram
    evaluation of, 129
bladder infections. *See* urinary tract infection
    (UTI)
bladder neck contracture
    post radical prostatectomy, 65
    treatment options for, 81–82
bladder outlet obstruction brachytherapy/inter-
    stitial seed therapy-related, 68
bladder ultrasound/scanner for PVR, 124, 126
bleeding
    during prostatectomy, 61–62
    with TURP, 150
blood, in urine and ejaculate, 19
blood pressure, PDE-5 inhibitor effect on, 228
blood tests, for prostate cancer, 9
blood thinners, penile injection therapy
    and, 239
blood transfusion, during TURP, 151
bone metastases, 21–22
    IV medications for, 52
bone pain
    symptomatic, in prostate cancer, 18
    treatment of, 118–120
bone scan
    procedure, 34, 38
    in staging, 38–39
bowel changes, external beam radiation
    therapy-related, 74–75
BPH (benign prostatic hyperplasia)
    5-alpha reductase inhibitors for, 135,
        137–140
    alpha-blockers for, 133–137
    AUS symptom score for, 123, 125
    bladder ultrasound/scanner PVR
        determination, 124, 126
    causes of, 122
    combination therapy for, 140–141
    conditions which mimic, 130, 131
    cystoscopy, 126–127
    damage from, 131, 132
    defined, 4
    diagnosis of, 123–130
    digital rectal exam for, 123
    disorders mimicking, 130–131
    herbal therapy for, 144
    indications for treatment, 132
    medical therapies for, 133–144
    minimally invasive surgical procedures for,
        145, 151–159
    prevalence of, 122

surgical procedures for, 145–151
symptoms of, 5, 122–123
tests for diagnosis, 124, 126–130
urodynamic study, 127–130
uroflow measurement for, 124
brachytherapy/interstitial seed therapy, 46, 49
    adjunctive external beam radiation
        therapy with, 71
    candidate for, 70–71
    ED after, 77
    PSA increase following, 116–117
    PSA monitoring following, 71–72
    radioactive agents in, 67
    results of, 72
    side effects of, 67–68
    technique, 66–67
breast cancer mutation gene (BRCA1), as risk
    for prostate cancer, 19
breast swelling (gynecomastia), 108

C

cancer, defined, 10
Cancer Risk Calculator for Prostate Cancer,
    13–14
carcinoma in situ of bladder, mimicking
    BPH, 131
cardiac status, interaction with PDE-5
    inhibitors, 224
cardiovascular risk, testosterone replacement
    therapy and, 212
Cardura (doxazosin), 134
Casodex (bicalutamide), 98, 100–101
catheterization, clean intermittent, 160–161
catheter(s)
    Foley, 68
    placement in radical prostatectomy, 55
    suprapubic, 68
        postoperative, 146
    urethral
        indwelling for BPH, 160
        postoperative, 146–148
    in urodynamic study, 128–129
Caverject. *See* intracavernous penile
    injection therapy
cavernosonography, for ED diagnosis, 194
chemotherapy
    for hormone refractory/resistant prostate
        cancer, 111–112
    for prostate cancer, 46, 51–52
chest pain, interaction with PDE-5
    inhibitors, 224
Chlamydia trachomatis, prostatitis from, 164
cholesterol levels, as cause of ED, 176–177
cholesterol-lowering drugs, as cause of ED,
    180–181
Chronic bacterial prostatitis, 161, 162
Chronic prostatitis/chronic pelvic pain
    syndrome, 162
Cialis (tadalafil), 209, 221–222, 225–226
clean intermittent catheterization
    for acute urinary retention, 68–69
    for BPH, 160–161

Index